Women's Cancers: Pathways to Healing

D0872865

J. Richard Smith

Women's Cancers: Pathways to Healing

A Patient's Guide to Dealing with Cancer and Abnormal Smears

Co-author: Giuseppe Del Priore

Illustrated by Dee MacLean

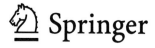 Springer

Authors
J. Richard Smith, MD, FRCOG
West London Gynaecological Cancer Centre
Imperial College at Hammersmith & Queen Charlotte's Hospitals
London, UK
Adjunct Associate Professor
New York University School of Medicine
NY, USA

Giuseppe Del Priore, MD, MPH
Vice President Research
NY Downtown Hospital
Associate Professor
Weil Medical College
Cornell University
New York, NY, USA

ISBN 978-1-84628-437-3   e-ISBN 978-1-84628-438-0
DOI 10.1007/978-1-84628-438-0

British Library Cataloguing in Publication Data
A catalogue record for this book is available from the British Library

Library of Congress Control Number: 2008934039

Cover illustration: Vladimirka Road, painted by Levitan in 1892. Reproduced with kind
permission of the Tretyakov Gallery, Moscow.

Printed on acid-free paper

Springer Science + Business Media
springer.com

This book is dedicated to all those women we have had the privilege to look after and who have encouraged the use of the 4-cusp approach and thus this project.

Preface

This book is designed, as the title "Pathways to healing" suggests, to allow you and your family ready access to all the information you require about your cancer to allow you to understand the different directions your disease may take. It should allow you to realize the breadth of possible outcome from where you stand at the particular point in time when you buy the book, or as your disease progresses or not. This book has been written for you wherever you are in the disease, ranging from cured, to those that spend many years living with their cancer, to those who sadly die of their cancer. One of the greatest privileges working in the field of cancer care is meeting many wonderful people, some of who have very kindly written sections of this book. We do hope that by reading this book things may be a little clearer for you and at least some worries made lighter.

J. Richard Smith
Giuseppe Del Priore

"Above all, what matters is not to lose the
joy of living for the fear of dying."

Maggie Keswick Jencks, Co-founder of Maggie's Cancer Caring Centres
By kind permission of Laura Lee CEO Maggie's

Acknowledgments

I would like to thank my wife, Deborah, for all her help and support through a long germination process. Thanks also to the late Roger Houghton, Nina Martin-Brown, and the late Ann Martin, literary agents without whose teaching, guidance, and encouragement this book would never have been produced. My sister Alison Reid was highly instrumental in allowing me the time to write this book. My thanks also go to Mr. Sam Abdalla, Mr. Shaun Hammond, Ms. Suzanne Thomas, Dr. Charles Innes, and the Rev. Gary Bradley, all of whom, over time, have shaped much of the thinking in this book. I met three people while on holiday who have been very helpful with this project and they are Father Vito Borgia and Joe and Carol Puttock. I would also like to thank Ms. Rodena Kelman, Mrs. Liz Lainis, and Ms. Vicky Lynch for all their secretarial support without which there would be no book. My thanks also go to Mrs. Pietraszewska, Sr. Catherine Gillespie, Mrs. Jo Abrams, and Dr. Mark Bower for reading the text and making many helpful suggestions. Mr. Tom Lewis and Dr. Bruce Barron have my gratitude for their friendship, support, and introduction to Dr. Del Priore.

Many of the pictures appeared in two-tone form originally in the "Patient Pictures" series published by Health Press and my thanks go to the publisher Sarah Redstone for allowing their reproduction again. Thanks also to Mr. Andy Nordin editor of Patient Pictures Gynaecological Oncology.

My thanks also go to Laura Lee and the Board of Maggie's Centres for allowing the use of the quote in the front fly leaf.

Finally, and last but certainly not least, I would very much like to acknowledge Dr. Giuseppe Del Priore, for his help, wise advice, and editorial skills; any mistakes and idiosyncrasies are mine.

About the Author

My name is Richard Smith and I am a Consultant Gynaecological Surgeon who specializes in treating women with cancer. I was born and educated in Scotland, graduating from Glasgow University (MB, ChB). I subsequently underwent postgraduate training in the West of Scotland and London. In the late 1980s, I worked at St. Mary's Hospital in London and did my thesis on the interaction of infections with cervical cancer (MD, Glasgow).

I have worked for many years the Chelsea and Westminster Hospital and have recently joined the new West London Gynaecological Centre at the Hammersmith Hospital in West London. In terms of Teaching, I am a Senior Lecturer at Imperial College School of Medicine, London, UK, and Adjunct Associate Professor at New York University School of Medicine.

I have had a long running interest in doctor–patient communication and have edited two series of books (The "Guide to …" series and another series, "Patient Pictures"), which were designed to help doctors and nurses explain surgical operations to their patients. These books have sold well (approximately 240,000 copies), suggesting that colleagues, both nursing and medical, are very much interested in this area, not what you would think from looking in the press!

I have always been keen on the synthesis of "standard" or orthodox medicine with "complementary" medicine. This started with being taught hypnosis, practicing it, and has subsequently widened out to include referring my patients for hypnotherapy, homeopathy, acupuncture, counseling, and psychotherapy. Over the last decade I have also become convinced that although I believe that people with some form of religious belief do not survive longer, I am sure they cope better with their cancer. For those with no religious sentiment there are other ways of helping them to find the inner self. The synthesis of these factors allows for a truly holistic approach.

My co-author, Giuseppe Del Priore is also a gynecologist specializing in cancer treatment. He works at New York Downtown Hospital, Weill-Cornell School of Medicine in New York City and has a long-standing interest in doctor–patient communication. He has been a pioneer in the field of fertility-sparing surgery.

The artist for the book is Ms. Dee MacLean, who is one of the foremost medical artists in the world today. She has an outstanding ability to make complex anatomy look comprehensible to both doctors and patients and has a long running interest in illustrating medical problems for patients. The Rev. Gary Bradley is the Vicar of the Churches of Little Venice, London, and Founder and Chairman of the Westminster Bereavement Council.

Mrs. Mira Dharamshi, Mrs. Patricia Walker, Mrs. Gallina Dean, and her husband John kindly wrote pieces as to their feelings about living with their cancer, or in John's case, his wife's cancer.

Contents

General Information

1. General Introduction

I have written this book in the hope of providing women who have been told that they have a cancer with accurate information that combines both orthodox medical treatments along with complementary therapies. I also hope it proves a valuable resource for families and supportive friends.

Compared to 20 years ago, there are now many sources of information available to patients. These range from a plethora of "mind, body, soul" books to innumerable web sites, many of which contain highly dubious, if not frankly wrong, information. In addition, you can, via 'Medline' or PubMed' services on the Internet, access precisely the same academic papers as the doctors and nurses who care for you. Unfortunately, these papers are not written in "patient-friendly" form.

The first goal of this book is to provide you with accurate information. The second goal is that I have always believed that a combination of "orthodox medicine" and complementary therapies, ranging from acupuncture to homeopathy, hypnotherapy, reiki, etc., allows people the best way through their diagnosis, treatment, and follow-up. I am a firm believer that all cancer patients deserve to hear the truth and that, contrary to popular belief, the truth, however painful, if properly imparted should not destroy hope. Below are what I would describe as the "golden rules."

The Golden rules of cancer management are:

1. Never say never. If you or your doctor believes that you are beaten before you start, then you are!
2. We should never say that there is nothing more that we can do for you – there always is!
3. The patient and the doctor are on the same team and should be working towards the same commonly understood and shared goals: quantity of life, but only if accompanied by quality.
4. I do not believe that spiritual peace necessarily increases longevity, but I do feel through many years of observation that those with it fare better in the cancer process than those without it. For those who have not explored this aspect of themselves, there are various ways in, some of which do not involve any religion.

How to Read the Book

This book is designed for you to read, more or less, from start to finish. It starts with four chapters which apply to all women diagnosed as having cancer. The next six chapters apply to each specific site of disease: cervix (neck of womb,) ovary, uterus (womb), vulva, breast, and choriocarcinoma (cancers relating to the afterbirth). Then follow chapters on chemotherapy and radiotherapy which will only be relevant to those undergoing that type of treatment. The chapters on pain management may not be relevant if you are not suffering from pain and you probably will not be. Most readers will want to read the sections on complementary therapies and spiritual approaches to living with cancer.

All readers should read Gary Bradley's chapter on bereavement because this does not as you might suppose just relate to death, but to the whole process of coming to terms with one's diagnosis and treatment. Inevitably for all, this will involve some loss, at its most minor this may be loss of that feeling of indestructibility, which we all tend to go through life with, to loss of organs etc. This chapter is therefore a "must read" for all.

Whenever I explain to my patients that they have a diagnosis of cancer, I always utilize the "4-cusp" approach. This seems to have proved very helpful to many women over the years, both to themselves and also in allowing them to explain to their families where they are in the process. The 4-cusp approach is really like a map for people with cancer. To facilitate its use, i suggest you draw the 4 cusps on a piece of paper so that you can mark on it where you feel yourself to be. It demonstrates that there is hope. There is nothing more important than hope. There are three groups who have hopes: you, your family, and your doctors and nurses. These hopes may vary and almost certainly will vary during the course of your disease whether you are cured or not. Hope is vital. Overall, in women with gynecological cancer over half get cured. For those who do not get cured, there is real hope of a number of years of good quality living. For those whose disease progresses, there is hope of excellent symptom control and comfort. For those who have sadly reached the end of their time, there is hope for peace and death without pain.

"Concept of Cure"

"Cure" naturally sits very high in people's thoughts, but there are many misconceptions about what makes one cancer more curable than another. In truth, it comes down to a number of factors including which organ the cancer is in, has it spread from that organ, is it removable surgically, is it sensitive to chemotherapy/radiotherapy, how strong/fit is the patient, and finally and most difficult of all to know, how "aggressive" is the tumor itself. We all know people who have had cancer that has "just run through them" in quick order and others who are never cured of their cancer but live with it for years. The difference between these two groups is often down the intrinsic aggressiveness of the tumor, something which is not easy to predict. This is why the wise doctor will avoid timespans.

You may or may not notice that there is no mention of statistics. This is because statistics apply to groups of patients, not individual patients. They do **not** help in trying to predict what will happen to **you.** The other thing people often think statistics will help with is answering the age-old problem of "how long have I got, doctor?" – they don't!

Telling people how long they have got is a very risky thing to start doing. Quite genuinely, your doctor will rarely know the answer to this question.

I do trust that you will find reading this book useful. The chapters have been contributed by colleagues and by three of my patients who felt very strongly that the 4-cusp approach had helped them. Sadly Mira, one of these three patients, has recently died. This was after having genuinely "lived" with her cancer for many, many years. She and many others have given me encouragement to write this book and we all hope that you get some good from it.

One final note, the cusps (A, B, C, D) are NOT in ANY way the same as "stages." The 4 cusps have proved useful to many patients, some have not found them useful, but the only people who have suffered from the concept are those who have got cusps mixed up with stages. All gynecological cancers are staged (I, II, III, IV). There is no relationship between stages and cusps – not even a wee bit!

2. Anatomy Overview

The Female Genital Tract

- The female genital tract includes the vulva, vagina, cervix, uterus, Fallopian tubes, and ovaries.
- The vulva is the area surrounding the openings of the vagina and urethra, which includes the clitoris.
- The vagina is a muscular tube that runs from the vulva to the cervix.
- The cervix, which is sometimes called the neck of the womb, is quite firm and lies at the bottom of the uterus. During labor, it softens and then opens to allow the baby to be born.
- The uterus is a muscular organ, usually about the size of a pear, that sits in the pelvis. It is here that the fetus develops during pregnancy. The lining of the uterus is called the endometrium. This thickens during the menstrual cycle in preparation for a fertilized egg, and is shed during menstruation if the egg is not fertilized.
- The two ovaries sit on either side of the uterus. In addition to producing eggs, they produce the female hormones, estrogen and progesterone, until menopause occurs.
- The fallopian tubes connect the uterus to the ovaries. When an egg is released from one of the ovaries, it is collected by the fallopian tube. Once in the tube, it may be fertilized by a sperm that has swum up from the vagina though the cervix and uterus.

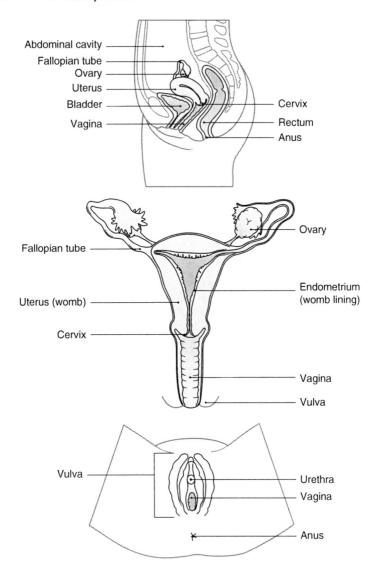

The Lymphatic System

- Lymph vessels are very fine tubes that drain the fluid called lymph, which escapes into the body's tissues. They run next to the arteries and form a network that returns the watery fluid into the bloodstream near the heart.

- Lymph nodes, sometimes called glands, are swellings that occur near the main arteries. They act as filters for the lymph, and also have a role in the body's immune system.
- Microscopic cancer cells can escape into lymph, and can become trapped in lymph nodes. If the cells then grow, they form growths called metastases. This is one of the common ways that many cancers can spread to different parts of the body.
- Surgery for many types of cancer (including cervical, endometrial, and vulval cancers) usually involves removing lymph nodes and the nearby lymph vessels.

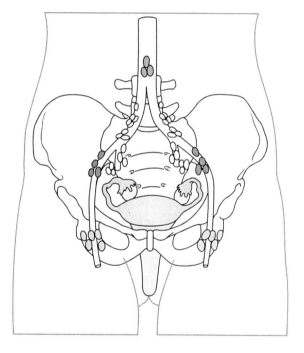

Pelvic and groin lymph nodes

Para-aortic nodes

Common iliac nodes

Internal iliac and obturator nodes

External iliac nodes

Inguinal (groin) nodes

3. The 4-cusp Approach to Cancer Care

My colleagues, medical oncologist Dr. Mark Bower and specialist nurse Sr Catherine Gillespie, and I have developed this approach to patient care over many years of sitting in clinics explaining to patients where they are with their cancer, not just in physical terms but conceptually in relation to their cancer and their life expectancy and its quality. Do draw the "4 cusps" so that you can use the model and mark on it where you are.

IT IS VITALLY IMPORTANT TO STATE THAT THE "4 CUSPS" (A–D) BEAR NO RELATIONSHIP TO THE FOUR STAGES (I, II, III, IV) OF CANCER.

Stages refer to how far a cancer has spread and are described in detail in Chapters 5–9.

Perhaps the two most important aspects of the model are the action of folding it down the central line and the "circle" aimed at in both cusps A and B. I believe that being able to fold the paper and thus dispatch cusps C and D to being "out of sight," coupled with the powerful image of a circle suggesting "holism," is the model's strongest features. This pictorial representation or 'map' to having cancer has seemed to resonate with patients and their families. Perhaps symbols can represent concepts that are difficult to explain with language. In the words of St. Thomas Aquinas, "man cannot understand without images."

When you are told of your cancer diagnosis, you will probably jump to the conclusion that you have been given a "death sentence." You will almost certainly immediately forget the remainder of the consultation, and only remember the diagnosis itself. The first thing I am able to tell the vast majority of my patients is that they are not in cusps C and D, and thus either in cusp A or B, and thus we can fold the paper down the dotted line and that we can literally put cusps C and D out of the way. You may find it helpful to do this right now with the "4 cusp you have drawn."

All of us are different and every cancer is different, but it is important in the first instance to be aware that *over 50% of gynecological tumors are cured in the long term*. The "death sentence" outlook is just not true for most people. At your first consultation for a suspected or confirmed cancer you will be given an outline of the timetable as to when investigations will be done and, if necessary, when and where your surgery will take place. You will be told that full results including exactly how far your cancer has progressed will be known by a specific date. At that time it will be possible to talk far more accurately about your outlook and prospects. The specific timetable to confirm the diagnosis, undertake any surgery, and obtain the results of the analysis of the removed cancer should take 2–4 weeks approximately, although this may be quicker (1 week) for some and slower (5–6 weeks) for others.

When all the information is available your doctor will wish to talk to you, perhaps on the ward or more often in a consultation room. Your doctor will tell you your results and what these will mean for you. My own golden rule here is to impart the truth, and nothing but the truth, in as gentle a fashion as possible. More and more doctors are receiving training in communication and it is likely that the appropriate language will be used. Sadly, but not surprisingly, it is known that this type of doctor–patient communication is the greatest cause of anxiety for doctors in training. Inevitably, however much training people have, some prove better at it than others. It is a facet of human nature that all of us prefer to tell people good news and most of us generally shy away from bad news, either giving or receiving it. All the professional training that goes into creating doctors cannot, nor for that matter should it, negate these emotions. We all know that in our daily lives we meet people whom we describe as "sensitive" or "insensitive," and this applies as much to doctors as to their patients. It is also true that in terms of personality type, the person who chooses to become a surgeon tends to be at the more self-confident and aggressive end of the spectrum, which are not features that always predispose to "touchy feely" behavior, but they do, however, tend to make for bold and effective surgeons.

The other factor that comes into play is the "dynamic" of the relationship between two individuals. Forgetting the medical situation, we all know that when we walk into a party where we do not know many people, in general, we will get along OK with most people, sometimes we will become good friends with somebody we meet, and occasionally we might marry that good friend. The opposite sometimes happens where we meet somebody we truly dislike. It is worth remembering that they probably feel the same way about us! The nature of human relationships is that although "we feel for ourselves," these feelings are usually mutual and reciprocated.

The professional relationship between patient and doctor is designed to remove the extremes described above (doctors who hate or marry their patients tend to end up not being doctors!), but it does not detract from the fact that we all still get on better with some people than with others. A good doctor should have the sensitivity and capacity to get on with the vast majority of his/her patients.

A commonly asked question is: "How long have I got?" No doctor is likely, if he/she has any sense, to answer this question directly, since they do not and cannot know the answer. They are much more likely to answer using a variant of my 4-cusp approach to cancer care. This is patient-centered and allows you to see where you are with your disease. I have spent many years drawing pictures for patients, showing them which operation they are going to have. Rarely has the picture been taken away for future reference. This may be because of the quality of my artwork or it may be that people get the message. On the other hand, the "4-cusp" diagram has been taken away by numerous patients who have found it very helpful, both for themselves and to assist in further dialogue with their families.

Cusp A	Cusp B	Cusp C	Cusp D
Cured	Living with cancer	Preterminal	Terminal
Weeks–years	Months–years	Weeks–months	Hours–days

This has proved a very useful method of communicating concepts of cure, living and dying with cancer, and I will now explain it in more detail. This concept will be used throughout the book, so please read this section with care. It may be helpful to bookmark it.

The first cusp (cusp A) probably applies to you from the time of your first visit to the clinic, when your surgeon gives the likely diagnosis and discusses with you the plan of action to determine how advanced your cancer is and hopefully how to remove it. I am usually confident before surgery that I can either cure the cancer with surgery or, failing that, at least put you in the best jumping-off point for further treatment. It is unusual before surgery for me, or any other surgeon, to feel that a cancer is not capable of having its course radically altered and made either potentially curable, or capable of remission. What you need is an honest appraisal of the possibilities along with a plan of action. This should include the date of surgery, length of time in hospital, and when the final results of tests will be available. All tissue samples go to the laboratory for testing (histopathology and cytopathology) and it is these results that absolutely determine the diagnosis and how advanced the cancer is. It is almost always possible to achieve these results within 2–6 weeks of your first visit to the clinic. You and your family will therefore have a good idea of where you stand by a specific date in the near future.

Your surgeon will explain how much your cancer has spread (or not). This will determine whether you require no other treatment because you are thought to be cured or whether you may need radiotherapy or chemotherapy or a combination of the two, either just to be on the safe side or because a cure is not likely without them. In general, if surgery alone is the only treatment you will be told that you are highly likely to be cured. This, however, can only be confirmed by the passage of time and the longer all remains well, the higher is the likelihood that you will be cured. Your surgeon will rightly be buoyant and optimistic with you. He/she will however explain that there is a small chance of the cancer coming back (a relapse) and you will need to be seen in the clinic for a number of years. You fall into the following 4-cusp picture (Figure 3.1).

The following are case histories of patients, all of which directly relate to women I have looked after over the last few years and which illustrate my 4-cusp approach.

Patient 1. A 35-year-old woman is referred to the gynecology oncology clinic with bleeding after sex and her general practitioner suspects she may have a cervical cancer (remember the vast majority of women with bleeding after sex do not have cervical cancer). When I examine the woman I find a small cervical cancer with no evidence of spread elsewhere. I explain that I think she has a cancer, which has only developed recently and that I believe her to be highly curable by surgery alone. The patient is then admitted and I perform an examination in the theater with the patient asleep, in other words

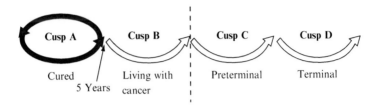

Figure 3.1. Cusp 'A'

under general anesthetic. This allows me to properly assess (see page 48) the tumor without any discomfort to the woman. This confirms that surgery is the best way forward and a few days later I perform a special type of hysterectomy (see page 50). One week later all the results are available.

Option 1: It is shown that the cancer has been completely removed and that there is no spread to the lymph nodes (glands). This means that the woman is presumed cured, i.e., she remains at **cusp A**.

Option 2: The tumor is completely removed but the cancer has spread to three lymph glands. I explain that these cancers do, if they are going to spread, tend to go to the lymph glands first. The lymph glands normally help to protect the body from infection, by acting as a kind of filter. When there is a cancer they also filter out cancer cells and prevent spread more widely through the body, so that although it is better not to have spread to the lymph glands, they have still done their job by preventing more extensive spread. In this woman's case the lymph glands have been removed, but because they have tumors in them she requires further treatment in the form of radiotherapy. I explain that this is probably overcautious, but still worthwhile (the "belt and braces" approach). This patient has entered **cusp B**: she is probably cured, but may not be, and is therefore "living with her cancer," certainly not dying of it. I also tell this woman to look in the mirror, and see herself: it is completely obvious that she is not looking at someone who is dying because she looks normal!

In terms of the 4-cusp model this is shown below. You may find it helpful to copy this onto your "4-cusp pullout."

4 Cusps

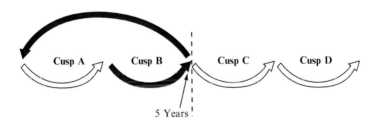

Patient 2. A 55-year-old woman goes to see her doctor since she has noticed swelling in her tummy over the last few weeks. She is referred to me and I agree that she seems to have a growth in her ovary. I explain that she may have a benign tumor or it may be malignant. Either way, she requires an ultrasound scan, a computed tomography (CT) scan, and some blood tests. The results of these tests suggest that she has a cancer within her ovary, but it appears to be confined to one ovary with no spread (this is called Stage 1, see page 53). It is explained to the woman that she requires surgery in the form of a hysterectomy and removal of both ovaries (see page 56), lymph nodes (glands), and a fatty structure in the abdomen called the omentum (see also page 56). I have never yet had a patient (unless they were a doctor themselves) who has heard of the omentum. I always explain that this fatty structure moves around the abdomen to where there is trouble. For example, in the past (pre-1900), before surgery was widely available, if you had an appendicitis you were quite likely to die; however, you could be saved by your omentum, which would move round the appendix and stop the infection spreading. Unfortunately, the omentum also moves itself around ovarian cancers to prevent them from spreading, but in the process cancers easily spread to the omentum itself; hence, we like to remove it. I have never met a woman who has missed her omentum once it is out! One week later the patient undergoes the planned operation.

Option 1: A tumor is removed, which is in one ovary alone. The patient requires no further treatment and is presumed cured; in other words, she is in **cusp A** as shown in Figure 3.2. Five years later she remains in remission and the inverted commas have been removed. She is cured and has entered the "cured circle".

Option 2: The patient is found to have cancer in both her ovaries and fluid containing cancerous cells in her abdomen. She requires chemotherapy: she has entered **cusp B.** It is explained that she has good prospects for cure, but that only time will confirm this: she is "living with cancer." However, 5 years later she has shown no sign of tumor recurrence and therefore has returned to cured status (the cured cirlce). This is shown in Figure 3.3.

Option 3: The patient is found at surgery to have disseminated (or widespread) cancer all over her abdomen. The technical term for how far the cancer has spread is the "stage" of the cancer, in other words, how advanced it is, and in this case it is called Stage 3 (see page 53). She is now in **cusp B.** It is explained that chemotherapy can be expected to work, but it cannot be said with certainty how great will be the effect. Some cancers respond extremely well to chemotherapy, some poorly, and the majority somewhere in between. Thus, it may not

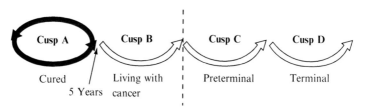

Figure 3.2. Cusp A. The Cured Circle

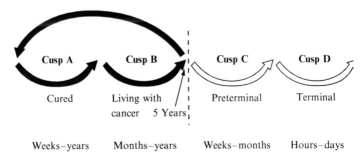

Figure 3.3. Return to cusp A. The Cured Circle

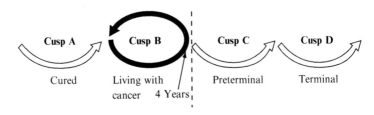

Figure 3.4. The Living with Cancer Circle

produce a cure; however, the longer it keeps the tumor under control, the better it is, both directly in terms of possible cure and indirectly, since the tumor that responds to chemotherapy in the first instance is more likely to respond to a second course of treatment. Thus there are three scenarios here:

(a) Excellent response and at 5 years the patient has no sign of tumor recurrence; thus, she has returned to **cusp A** (see Figure 3.3).

(b) A good response is found and the patient remains well for 4 years, at which point she develops recurrence of her cancer. She is treated again with the same chemotherapy as before with good prospects of similar 2–4-year response. Thus she remains in **cusp B** (see Figure 3.4).

(c) A poor response is observed, with the cancer recurring 4 months later. This patient has now entered **cusp C** (see Figure 3.5).

This woman has very little chance of cure and has therefore entered the pre-terminal phase of her illness. She is informed that she is unlikely to be cured and that she has a limited time left to her, which may be weeks or months, but is unlikely to be longer than this. She is informed that there are plenty of treatment options still available, and although these are designed mainly to enhance quality of life, they may also extend it. These types of treatment are called palliative care and may include pain relief, treatment of constipation or diarrhea, and many other aspects that are described in Chapter 13.

Three of my patients kindly agreed to write a piece for this part of the book because they felt strongly that they had very much benefited from the concept of "living with cancer." Sadly, Mira, one of them, has recently died and I have

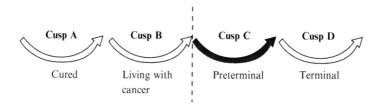

Figure 3.5. The "Pre-terminal cusp"

therefore followed her wishes, namely of publishing the piece unedited. This was her specific request and I have to say that while the sentiments expressed in her piece are very flattering to me, I suggested that they would be better not appearing in print! Mira told me that she wished them printed as she had written them and I have therefore followed her wishes and not exercised any editorial control!

Healing – What Role Can Faith Play?

I remember clearly the day I was told I had ovarian cancer. My first thoughts were: Why me? What have I done wrong? Not that I was a stranger to cancer, having lost a younger sister to the disease several years earlier. She was diagnosed with leukaemia, so I was well versed with the 'Big C'. I had seen her go through the trauma of chemotherapy and radiotherapy. But only in hindsight do I realise that I experienced for the first time the role that faith could play in helping one cope with the illness. At the time, I would ask my sister cynically: Where is God now that you need him most? Her reply was always that God was giving her the strength to go through this. In my wisdom then, I required proof of God's existence because if he existed, why wasn't he helping her?

Proof of course is beside the point. The essential issue for me now is 'faith'. It is, I believe, the driving force behind my ability to persevere through my cancerous journey. Faith can take many guises: faith in God or some sort of spiritual plane; faith in oneself, one's consultant, one's family, friends etc. My own faith takes many forms.

My faith can certainly be summed up as a conventional belief in God. But my consultant, medical treatment, and support and help from people around me also play an important role in my well being.

I felt extremely angry watching my sister go through her illness. But her courage and faith that she would ultimately get better never wavered. Unfortunately she passed away a few months later. I promised myself that if I ever developed cancer, I wouldn't go through what she had, that is, the gruelling treatment in a bid to extend the amount of time I had. How wrong was I, as here I am, after many years of living with and tackling the disease, telling my tale.

I did want to die as soon as I was told that I had cancer. My reasoning was that I could escape the pain and suffering through early release.

After receiving news about my illness from the doctor, I remember vividly standing at a bus stop. It was New Year's Eve, the streets were full of Christmas decoration, crowds were rushing about and it was bitterly cold. I didn't know whom to talk to. My husband was at work; should I tell him immediately or wait until I knew the prognosis? I stood zombie-like, numb – my mind scheming and plotting some sort of plan on what to do next. Having no other immediate family in London except for my husband, I felt alone. I wanted to spare him the anguish I felt seeing my sister go through her illness. I would be dead soon, I thought. But what would happen to my husband and my nieces? And, in the meantime, how would I tell my father, who lived in Kenya? The shock, I thought, may kill him.

As it turned out, I was spared the decision of telling my father news of my illness as he passed away in the interim period before my consultant's appointment. I also refrained from telling my family and made an excuse not to attend my father's funeral. Understandably, the family considered this odd as I was viewed as his favourite daughter and supported him financially.

I decided I would visit the consultant alone. After all, I knew exactly what I wanted: in the event that the disease was substantial, I didn't want any treatment at all – such was my lack of faith in myself, medicine and ultimately God.

The first appointment was a mixed bag; the consultant was very smart, looked very young, I was told by my gynaecologist that he was the best. And now I know he is, nevertheless, he was very amenable to talk to. He explained in detail that I had a lump on my Inferior Vena Cava and a 'mass' on my ovary. A hysterectomy was therefore on the cards.

I was devastated by the prognosis. I could feel tears rolling down my cheeks despite the fact I had promised myself I wouldn't break down. But I was comfortable talking to him, describing how I felt and telling him about my sister. I didn't want any treatment if the cancer was widespread and definitely no chemotherapy. After lengthy discussions with my consultant, it was agreed that he would undertake an exploratory operation to assess the situation, and then discuss the way forward. He agreed, though, to respect my wishes and would do whatever I decided.

The trials that followed over the next seven years included: five operations; three sets of chemotherapy of carboplatin, Taxol, radiotherapy; contracting septicaemia; losing my hair, accompanied by fun and games with wigs and turbans; and, unrelated to the illness, breaking my right arm, which resulted in the insertion of two metal pins and a plate in my elbow, having a younger brother gunned down by a bank robber in Nairobi. In addition, I almost lost the one thing I continue to enjoy immensely – my job – after the company underwent one of the most acrimonious and hostile take-overs ever fought in the City of London. Being told my job no longer existed was an enormous shock and filled me with the dread of having to find another job – an almost impossible task, I thought, given my medical history. For the time being I have managed to secure a position in the Marketing Department, but for how long?

At one point, a nurse had said to me: "I have seen you down in the dumps many times, but you always pick yourself up. I don't know how you do it?" Similarly, I don't know what drives me to persevere, despite the difficulties associated with the illness as well as life's hardships. Sometimes, I wonder that I am from another planet and am an alien, it is just not possible all these things happening, seems like a James Bond movie drama despite going through hell and fire you, come out smiling.

My colleagues have sometimes joked that the sickness record in the office has dropped as a result of my attitude. If I can make it to the office whilst undergoing chemotherapy, for example, they can also show up for a day's work even when they have minor ailments. But I don't necessarily entertain a positive attitude – despite others' belief to the contrary – and have never been afraid of dying. My aim is to maintain a good quality of life, not to live at any cost and be a burden to my family.

It is difficult to express what drives me; perhaps it is just sheer determination. I manage to hold a full-time job, tackling the daily commute into and out of London by changing two trains, and often working late into the evening. I have continued working daily while having chemo and, at one point, had to contend with one arm in plaster for eight weeks.

Waiting for a bus one day, I overheard a lady say: "O' it was God sent." This struck a cord with me. God may not touch you directly, but someone or something in your life can give you strength – be it your general faith, husband, a friend, a nurse, or ones faith in a consultant.

The thing I most remember is my consultant saying to me that I should allow him to help rid me of cancer. He also expressed hope that I could avoid the thing I dreaded most – chemotherapy. His words proved powerful. He said he would give his sister, for example, exactly the same advice if she were in the same position as me. This ultimately prompted me to change my mind and agree to have the exploratory operation and the subsequent treatment. Here was someone I didn't know, wasn't related to me, but cared for me and wanted to help make me better. He listened to my concerns, explained in detail that I was in the so-called second cusp – that is, living with cancer – and exactly how he planned to treat me. I would never ask him how long I had as I think no one can give you that guarantee.

The upshot is that deep in my inner self, the faith I have in God gives me strength. Many a times I ask God: "Why am I being punished? What have I done? I consider myself to be a good person, but not a saint. I often recall what my mother used to say when questioned about God and different aspects of worship. "I am your mother, a wife to your father, an aunt, a grandmother, a daughter, but I am only one person. God also has numerous names, but is only one. No one has seen him; though we all believe that he exists and have faith that he will provide strength in times of need."

Travelling to work each day – which takes roughly over one hour – I recite my prayers. I pray for world peace, for all who are sick and need help, pray that God gives me strength to cope with my illness and that I do not suffer or prove to be a burden to my family toward the end of my illness. I also pray that, whenever it arrives, I meet a peaceful end.

Mira Dharamshi

This second piece has kindly been written by Patricia Walker.

I must have been living with cancer a long while before finding out. I did not even connect a series of rather vague symptoms, ranging from repeated bouts of cystitis to an increasingly swollen stomach. When I appeared, to me at least, to look in an advanced state of pregnancy, the duty GP simply asked if I had considered liposuction. Eventually sudden breathtakingly sharp stomach pains sent me to hospital.

The diagnosis of Stage 3 ovarian cancer, and the subsequent removal of "a tumour the size of a rugby ball" two days before my 64th birthday, was a complete and potentially devastating surprise. I had no real idea of what it meant and found it hard at first to absorb the information I was given. Happily, almost as big a surprise was the number of ways that the hospital team helped me to cope. I was important that from the very beginning, like others on the gynaecological ward, I was treated not just as a patient, or a case, or a hospital number, but as a named individual whose personal concerns and preferences were sought, considered and taken into account.

Doctors have something in common with airline pilots. They have to strike a balance between being seriously knowledgeable and competent and being reassuringly relaxed, and to do this without sounding so laid back and blasé that their passengers (patients) expect the worst. I liked the tone of voices at the C&W very much: realistic, warm, comforting, professional, personal.

The Gynaecology Consultant was extraordinarily generous with his time, explaining the diagnosis, proposed operation, likely treatment and intended outcome. He drew annotated diagrams which, if not high art, very effectively communicated the facts and have been invaluable for later reference. The Oncologist knew that my husband had been a patient at the C&W and thoughtfully took this into account with options for treatment. The supporting professionals also communicated well, listening and responding to what they were being asked. The different disciplines involved in my treatment seemed to work as a cooperative and accessible team and me feel, at least temporarily, a part of that team and sharing the same focus.

My main reaction to all this was to feel personal responsibility for my progress and only a distant academic interest in discouraging statistics. I was not avoiding reality but deciding that all available energy would be needed for getting better.

Landmarks became very important. At first they were small and frequent: getting out of bed, coping without a catheter, having a shower (thank you, Sharon!), walking down the corridor. Every one was substantial reassurance that things were progressing as predicted. Later each chemotherapy treatment was a landmark, with the Ca125 blood test result assuming enormous significance and regularly demonstrating progress.

The biggest (to me) early landmark provided a salutary lesson: use landmarks, but don't depend on them. It was the joint Oncology/Gynaecology review booked before I left hospital. When neither consultant was available at the appointment (for very good reasons), the disappointment was like a physical blow.

By contrast, there was a positive physical effect from the consistent kindness, consideration, competence and cheerfulness found throughout the hospital. The Medical Day Unit where chemotherapy is administered is a particularly good example. Chemotherapy is not normally the jolliest way to pass a day but the staff have created a unique atmosphere and relationships with their customers, as well as their colleagues, that inspire confidence and give invaluable practical and psychological support and inspired confidence.

The first chemotherapy treatment, with carboplatin and taxol, had three particular side effects. One was hair loss which proved much less of a physical and emotional problem than anticipated. A wig, a knitted hat and two silk scarves covered every eventuality. The hair started growing back as soon as the chemotherapy finished. This was totally fascinating for my small granddaughters. My hair was the same colour – not always the case – but initially Afro-curly; then looser curls; then wavy as before chemotherapy; then straight.

A second side effect was the constipation, which did not go away. Experimenting with a variety of prescription medicines identified the most suitable, with prunes or prune juice and dried figs playing a major supporting role. The Medical Day Unit nurses were very familiar with the problem and their experience was invaluable.

A third side effect was neuropathy: numbness of the fingers and feet. Once the chemotherapy had finished, the fingers recovered fairly quickly; dipping them in alternatively hot and cold water helped. The balls of the feet and the toes did not. The nurses suggested treatment by a hospital based reflexologist, a trained therapist who volunteered her services one day a week. Reflexology every two or three weeks restored a great deal of feeling and made walking safer and more confident. It was also wonderfully relaxing. Other treatments available included massage and relaxation classes. While complementary therapies have their place and undoubtedly have been helpful to me, and how and where they are given is important. It proved quite impossible to learn relaxation techniques in an airless room on a carpet sprinkled with biscuit crumbs and discarded food wrappings.

Away from the hospital, I had two opportunities for Reiki treatments. The first one was remarkable. A warm glow over my stomach, although the practitioner had not touched me, produced complete relaxation and a sense of peaceful well being. The other had the opposite effect. The second practitioner talked non stop throughout about her own activities and plans for practising other therapies which left me twanging with tension.

During the first chemotherapy both my neighbour and sister in law had asked for remote spiritual healing for me. It was as important that they felt they were doing something to help as that I felt supported by them in this way. Coping with cancer can be as hard or harder for family and friends as for the patient, especially when they feel powerless. Individuals found so many ways to help: scouring the internet for information, recommending books they had enjoyed, sharing funny newspaper cuttings, cheerful telephone calls, not just inviting me to lunch or dinner but thoughtfully arranging transport too, and encouraging business as usual in terms of work.

Work has been as important as treatment. It has confirmed that my brain still works, that people still want to use it and that I still have something important to contribute. Getting paid is a very welcome endorsement of this. Equally important, however, has been the reassurance of a variety of charitable and other organisations which are just as eager for involvement and advice, even if more may be done by e mail or over the telephone than previously. Two new appointments while living with cancer have been particularly welcome, as both organisations were fully aware of the circumstances when they employed me.

How much people want to know differs. Sometimes "how are you?" expects a fairly detailed answer about treatment and response to it. For others" doing well" may be as much as they feel they can cope with. My daughter wants to know everything and from the first I made sure my medical notes said she was to be told everything.

It was ten months before I started chemotherapy again, this time with Caelyx. There was no hair loss, no sickness, no side effects, which suggested to me that it was having no effect. It was stopped after three cycles. Subsequently the Ca125 tests demonstrated an improvement.

It was at this stage that a group of close friends organised a marvellous event. Twenty female friends sat down to a lunch for which they had brought food, wine, flowers and much crockery. Many had never met each other before (but a lot of them have met again since). The premise was that all the compliments that are paid at funerals and memorial services are not heard by the one person they directly concern. So why not arrange a lunch where friends can pay their compliments in person? My daughter thought it sounded morbid but in the event she found it an incredibly happy, noisy and uplifting occasion- as I did – and she recorded the proceedings on video to prove it. It was a tremendously supportive and confidence inspiring day; and confidence – in the hospital, professionals, treatment, advice, information and people is the most important single aid to living with cancer.

Nearly three years after my operation, I was due to start chemotherapy again. The start was delayed: firstly because I was taking antibiotics for an infection, then for no apparent reason, despite a very high Ca125 result. It was a couple of months before affected patients were told that the National Health Service had decreed that all gynaecological cancers were to be treated at Cancer Centres and the Chelsea and Westminster had been designated a unit not a centre. We were compulsorily evicted from the hospital and from the team we knew and trusted. This was inevitably demoralising.

The Cancer centre has struggled to cope with the sudden influx of new patients at different stages of diagnosis and treatment. There were inevitable delays for the first appointment. It was months before chemotherapy started again, by then with a bigger job to do. Fortunately after the first two cycles the Ca125 has fallen dramatically and although the CT scan appears to show that the tumours have not shrunk, they are not noticeably larger.

In the bigger, busier specialist Cancer Centre there is not the same close team and continuity of staff. Although no doubt in excellent hands, those hands are constantly changing and it is much harder to establish relationships, not helped by the fact that surgeon and oncologist are now in different centres. It will therefore take a while to recover the confidence which is so essential to living with cancer.

The third piece has been written by Galina Dean and her husband, John.

SO FAR SO GOOD

One person's fight against Ovarian Cancer

In September 2002, at the age of 38, after 6 weeks of unexplained abdominal pain I was diagnosed with stage 4 Ovarian Cancer.

I had always thought of myself as a healthy person, with the exception of the fact that I had a benign ovarian cyst and the relevant ovary removed in 1982.

I had yearly ultrasound tests and internal examinations.

I felt that my health was good. I exercised regularly and had a good diet. My parents were both healthy and I did not imagine that anything serious could happen to me.

Looking back, I remember exactly when the symptoms started – it was in the middle of July 2002. My husband, John, and I had just returned from vacation in France. I constantly had a problem with constipation over 4–5 years but it got worse when we came back from vacation.

I had taken laxatives from time to time over a long period but increased the dosage after the holiday. The pain I experienced with any bowel movement was unimaginable. I also started having stomach spasms after eating and my abdomen became swollen.

I originally thought that this was a consequence of food poisoning in France. However, after a week the problem did not go away and so I went to see my local GP. He sent me home, saying that it was certainly food poisoning, and that I would be fine in a week or so.

I did not get better and went to see him again after 10 days.

By this time my abdomen was noticeably swollen and I was wearing the biggest trousers I had in my wardrobe.

He said, "I cannot see any problem, you look fine!" I said to him, "what do I have to do as I am having intense pain". He gave me pain killers and sent me home!

Within 4–5 days I was forced to queue up to see another doctor at the same practice who, after an internal examination organized a ultrasound test for me at the Chelsea & Westminster Hospital.

The girl in the Ultrasound room told me that there was nothing suspicious, and that I should come back in 2–3 months time.

At the time I asked her to look a little higher up in the stomach area, however she refused, saying that in the instruction from the GP the only request had been for an ultrasound of the ovary!

This was exactly one week before I was diagnosed with OVARIAN CANCER!!

The pain became more and more intense. I couldn't eat anything, my stomach was distended as if I was pregnant. I again went back to the original GP and begged him to organise a blood test. He said that this was not necessary as he now knew exactly what the problem was.

He sent me to the Lydia Clinic which at the time did not mean anything to me, and I went along with no misgivings.

The pain was so bad that I could hardly think about anything. However, imaging my surprise when I found out that this was a Venereal Disease Clinic!

My husband was very angry when I told him what had happened and attended the meeting the next day with the GP. We both insisted that he take a blood sample which he finally agreed to do.

That night I had a high temperature, had not eaten for 3-4 days and had difficulty breathing. The next morning I could not wait any more and asked my husband to take me to the hospital as an emergency case. The Chelsea & Westminster Hospital ("C&W") is no more than 10 - 15 minutes drive from our house and as we were driving there my GP called to say that he had the blood test results which were very bad and that we should go immediately to see him.

We did this and he gave us the paperwork for me to be admitted to the C&W as an emergency case.

There is an important point to be made here which is that:

If you suspect a problem which does not go away, be active and do not be "fobbed" off by your GP!!

In the worst case you can always pay for a blood test and take the results to your doctor. If I had known what I know now, I would have had a Ca125 test (tumour marker) done immediately. At the time I did not know that this kind of test existed. The normal range for this test is 0–23. At the time of my admittance my "score" was 2,700!!

I was admitted to C&W on a Friday and finally, after a full day of tests, I was given an MRI scan. I was then kept in hospital over the weekend whilst they drained the fluid which had been distending my abdomen.

Finally, the initial nightmare ended and on the Monday Mr Smith, the Gynaecological Surgeon, came to see me and told me that I had tumours on my ovary, my omentum and my stomach. He said that they had tested the fluid with which I was swollen to find that it was full of cancer cells. I also had fluid in my lungs.

Even though "cancer" was the last name I wanted to hear, I felt some relief that my illness at last had a name and I could start receiving treatment, and that maybe, one day, I would start feeling better.

I believed in Mr Smith, his kind eyes radiated confidence, and I knew that this man would help me.

John was there with me. No need to describe our feelings. We could not believe what was happening. This was something unreal. At this stage all I knew about cancer was that people died from it.

"Am I dying?" was my first question to Mr Smith. "How long do I have?" He explained that I was not in the terminal stage, so I had some time …

Then for my second question I asked Mr Smith to give me survival statistics for my situation. He said, "I will give you statistics if you want, but everybody is an individual case. Most women with the disease are over the age of 55".

I wanted to know anyway.

The answer was that only one in three to four women in the sample survived beyond 5 years. I could not believe what I was hearing. I was not ready. When Mr Smith's team left the room, John and I hugged one another and started crying together. …I felt that it was my fault that, because of my illness, I felt that I was letting him down, I was letting our relationship down and I was letting my parents and all my friends down.

That night I pulled myself together. I thought I had no right to let so many people down, so many people I loved, I could not let them suffer. I thought, "I will fight and I will survive".

On Mr Smith's recommendation and that of Dr Bower from the C&W Oncology Department, I had four rounds of chemotherapy (Taxol/ Carboplatin) before my operation. I had been warned about all the side effects. The worst one was that I was going to lose my hair, my long, blond hair, which I had always been proud of.

I was going to lose all of it…

I felt weak and helpless after the first round of chemo, I presumed in my case it was because I was having the treatment straight after being in hospital on a drip and "nil by mouth" for a week, so I was pretty weak already.

For the first 3–4 days after chemo, I lost weight, 1–1.5 kilos every day. My normal weight had been 50 kilos for the last 15 years and with the fluid accumulation it had reached 54. I felt very weak and tired, sometimes not to be able to lift a glass of water. It was pretty unpleasant, I felt like an invalid. I decided at that point to do something positive!!

Next morning I asked John to take me to the Ki Energy Institute in London, NW1. A close girl friend strongly recommended this approach. She had benefited enormously from their treatments and had been using them to boost her general health for 3 years. The method is derived from 6,000 year old Taoist tradition originating in South Korea. I could hardly walk, John almost carried me from the car.

After 2–3 hours of treatment, I felt much better, walking by myself and felt strong enough to walk in the park for 2 hours.

From that point I went there every day. For the first two weeks John drove me, and after that I was able to drive myself…I started to feel better from the first day and the pain lessened.

I did not take this for granted. I remember on bad days when I said to my husband, "If only this pain will go away, I will not ask for anything else, I will be the happiest person in the world!".

My weight stabilised around 48 kilos. The pain went completely and my stomach became flat again. I re-started a gentle exercise regime just to tone my muscles.

I bought a lot of books on the subject of cancer to investigate as much as possible. My first real inspiration came from the book, "The Cancer Battle", about a woman who was sent home to die with progressive breast cancer. 12 years on she is still alive, healthy and happy!

Reading this book, I realised that one has to take responsibility for one's own body.

The key statement in the book was "Your body has the ability to completely heal itself of any disease… all it needs is your assistance."

From this point the real action started:-

A reverse osmosis filter was installed in our house. Pure water is very important and with ovarian cancer I wanted to make sure that any oestrogen and any oestrogen mimics were removed from the water I was drinking.

I started to make fresh juice 3–4 times per day (carrot, apple, fennel, beetroot and wheat grass) this helps the body de-toxify. The concentrated amount of vitamins, minerals, enzymes in very fresh juice assimilate quickly and easily into one's blood. I stopped drinking coffee and tea, switching to herbal infusions/ teas. I gave up alcohol and stopped eating sugar, wheat, milk products and meat…

As soon as we found a sensible wig I had my hair cut off, (I still keep it as a souvenir), because the worst nightmare would have been to see my hair on the pillow every morning.

I realised very quickly that I had to make the best of the situation I was in, otherwise I would go mad. My wig was not cheap, but I rationalised this with the idea that I was going to save on shampoo, conditioner, haircuts, etc. for several months.

The rest of the rounds of chemotherapy went pretty well for me. I felt OK and managed to lead a more or less normal life, going out from time to time and going to the gym. I had been involved in the property market in a small way and was able to resume this activity.

I had my 4th round of chemo just before my birthday in November 2002. My Ca125 count was 32. On the 2nd December 2002 Mr Smith performed a hysterectomy and also removed my omentum.

After Christmas I had to face another 4 rounds of chemo, this finished in March 2003. Between rounds 6 and 7 of chemotherapy I visited the Paracelsus Klinic in Switzerland with my husband. I had talked to them a few weeks before and they had strongly suggested that this was a good time to be treated by them. Their approach is based on Biological Medicine, but the same time they try to work together with orthodox treatments. I had a very busy schedule and they performed many different tests on me. I was given a large box of pills to take every day with very little explanation.

I found it pretty stressful not to understand what I was being asked to put in my body. As I had a very low red blood cell count, I could not take all the treatments at that time. They therefore suggested that I come back after the last round of chemo, but it was a very, very expensive 2 weeks.

I wanted to make a clear plan of what I was going to do when the chemo finished. One of our friends gave a book entitled, "Everything you need to know to help you beat Cancer" by a biochemist, Chris Woollams. It is one of the most useful books that I have read.

He also gave me a copy of the magazine that Chris Woollams edits called, "ICON". I immediately subscribed to this magazine and have found it to be very useful.

The book contains a lot of information about how to help yourself recover after chemotherapy and tumour removal operations. I was shocked by the news that almost all cancer sufferers are very toxic, their bodies can be very acidic and can also have a high level of parasites, viruses and/or yeast.

So my first step was to check these things. I had all of them!

I met a woman at the Ki Energy Institute who had been diagnosed with melanoma 3 years ago. She had refused any orthodox treatment and had undertaken a course of natural healing instead. She recommended me to try Biotech Health in Petersfield, particularly a nutritionist called Anne Smitten. I think this was the wisest money I have spent on my way to recovery.

Food intolerance and vitamin/ mineral screening showed I could eat only fruit, vegetables, some grains and nuts. My body could not absorb any vitamins in tablet form. I had been taking just such tablets from the health store. Her tests showed that by doing this I was simply loading myself with even more toxins and making my liver work harder to digest all of it.

I went home with a clear plan for the next 6 months:

1. Detox
2. Diet
3. Nutrition
4. Coffee Enemas

As Anne likes to say, "One thing at a time. We have to be patient with you. When you get cancer, it means you have probably been doing something wrong for a long period of 3–5 years minimum so to fix it will take time as well. We have to get your body to change part of its chemistry".

I also had a hair analysis at the Wellbeing Clinic that showed a very high Mercury level in my body. So I found a holistic dentist to remove my amalgam fillings which can leak heavy metals into the body and overstretches the immune system. I had a special heavy metal detox programme after the fillings were removed.

In summer 2003, as part of my vacation, I visited the clinic in Moscow where Photodynamic Therapy (PDT) was created. They use what they call a photosensitise, a solution that is taken orally and when combined with laser light kills tumours. There are no cumulative toxic effects with PDT as with radiation and chemotherapy, so the procedure can be repeated several times if needed.

The Dove Clinic for Integrated Medicine offer this in the UK.

Dr Kenyon from the clinic recommended C-Statin for me. This is made from bindweed. The theory is that this contains inhibitors which stop the body from growing new blood vessels to supply tumours, which then cannot grow. Whilst I was in Russia I was introduced to Irina Filipova, Professor of Fungotherapy (Mushrooms). She tailor-made a plan for me, which included 5 types of mushrooms and some herbs. I have been taking this for one year now and have a great belief in it.

As I am in early menopause following my hysterectomy and have all the usual symptoms, I looked for a way to regulate my hot flushes and have found acupuncture to be of great assistance.

My Ca-125 is stable, within the normal range. I am enjoying life and every day is a special gift for me.

I would like to thank all the people who helped me through this very difficult time, especially my husband and all of the staff at the C&W particularly Mr J Richard Smith and Dr M Bower.

OVARIAN CANCER: A HUSBAND'S EXPERIENCE

Today is the fourth anniversary of the day on which I met my wife, Galina ("Gala"). In late summer 2002, without any warning, she was diagnosed with Stage 4 Ovarian Cancer at the age of 38.

In this circumstance one is immediately aware that the role of the husband is that of a supporting player in a drama where nature is in control.

We experienced both extremes of the National Health Service ("NHS") during the first 3 months:

The worst – anger and frustration at our GP's refusal to take my wife's symptoms seriously, seemingly more concerned about the use of NHS resources in requesting any tests which would have revealed the problem 5–6 weeks before it was finally discovered. This in light of the fact that Gala had an abdominal scar having had an ovary removed with a benign cyst 20 years earlier:

The best – First class care and attention at the hands of the Oncology team under Dr Mark Bower at Chelsea and Westminster Hospital and the Surgical Team under Mr J Richard Smith.

We will never know whether the delay has affected Gala's probability of survival. However, it is clear that without the help of the people at Chelsea & Westminster she would not be alive today!

Whilst being aware that Gala's body has to fight this problem, I have tried in my small way to make it a shared problem.

I believe that all husbands can make a difference in these circumstances. Whether or not it is admitted, anyone who is diagnosed with cancer is scared of dying and needs reassurance that there is always a chance of survival. One should be aware of the statistics but one should never accept that the worst outcome is inevitable.

I tried, wherever possible, to attend all meetings with Gala and to always drive her to the hospital and to which ever clinic she was attending. We went to Paracelsus Klinic in Switzerland together and I met with all of her doctors. I believe that it is important to try to retain a measure of control over one's own destiny, e.g. Gala knew that she would lose her long hair (a prized asset!) and so after the first treatment we found an understanding hairdresser, who gave her a No 1 cut and also advised on the purchase of a wig.

My advice is – do not be afraid to spend money on a good wig, even at the expense of some other seemingly necessary items. Nothing is more important at this time than maintaining self confidence and self esteem.

In Gala's case although she was extremely upset to lose her hair, she controlled the moment of loss herself. She also consoled herself with the knowledge that it was virtually certain to grow back stronger than ever.

I believe that the key is an open mind, a positive attitude and a determination to explore all avenues for treatment, both within traditional and non-traditional medicine. It seems to me that although brutal and toxic, chemotherapy and surgery are necessary evils. Galina has met a number of people who have only been prepared to undertake non-traditional solutions but in my opinion one reduces the probability for survival if traditional medical treatment is ignored.

I can only share with you our experiences and cannot say that this will work for everyone, but (fingers crossed) it is working for Gala. Her Ca 125 (tumour marker) numbers have gone from 2,700 before chemo to 7 as of today and are stable around this figure. (Normal range 0–23)

Anything that increases belief in survival has to be a good thing. It may be that some of the things that we have tried for Gala have simply increased her belief in her own survival rather than being effective in their own right. I do not think that this is the case but even if it was I would still go ahead with them. I am generally a sceptical person and I do not understand some of the treatments that she has received but I have seen the results with my own eyes.

After a course of chemotherapy one is faced with the fact that for a period no further treatments of this type can be undertaken for a long period. We therefore concentrated on 3 areas in looking for alternatives. We wanted to detox her body after the effects of the chemotherapy and also get rid of any heavy metals which could be inhibiting her immune system. We then concentrated on treatments that would generally boost her immune system. One of the first revelations for me was the fact that everyone produces cancerous cells continuously and one's immune system normally kills them.

Finally, we tried to find a treatment that would kill cancer cells without the toxic effects of traditional chemotherapy.

Gala has listed all the treatments that she has found to be useful. This may not be a comprehensive list and I would encourage everyone to explore all avenues to discover more diverse remedies. We could not find such a list when we started and it is entirely due to Gala's determination that we have covered the treatments mentioned. In conclusion this experience has brought us closer together.

We believe in the strategy that we have evolved for Gala and are grateful for each day. She is in remission and her tests are within the normal range. It is still early days and we cannot take anything for granted.

Commentary (by Richard Smith): Originally I had not intended to make any comment upon the pieces kindly written above. However having read them and digested them I have to say I find each deeply moving and all in different ways. It is purely by chance that all three patients should have adopted different strategies for coping with and handling their disease. It is important to say that there were no other pieces solicited which have subsequently been "spiked" (edited out) because they did not happen to suit. I am not able to comment upon many of the complementary therapies that Galina has described. Her piece does remind me of Michael Gerin-Tosh's very moving and important book, 'Living Proof – a Medical Mutiny.'

I do however believe that Galina whilst accessing a range of Complementary therapies has also rightly used the orthodox ones as well. John Diamond's book 'Snakedance' takes the opposite approach to Gearin-Tosh dismissing many complimentary therapies. As stated on many occasions in this book I personally believe that different strategies suit different patients and a combination of orthodox and complementary therapies are advantageous; the three pieces here amply demonstrate this. Finally I know that Galina and her husband feel very aggrieved by their General Practitioner and the failure to make an earlier diagnosis. This is very understandable.

I believe I should say, however, say that most patients with advanced ovarian cancer have usually taken some time to get diagnosed. This is not just down to incompetence but to the very real difficulty of making the diagnosis. The ovaries are not visible without sophisticated scanning, and the symptoms cancer on the ovary produces are often vague and difficult to interpret. This gives GPs and, for that matter, gynaecologists difficulties in making the diagnosis. The vexed subject of screening is covered on pages 52–53 which further elaborates on this difficult subject. I would, however, entirely concur with Galina that if you have persistent symptoms go back and let your doctor know.

We now return to examples of other patients.

Patient 3. A 60-year-old woman comes into the ward complaining of being unable to control urination. In fact she is permanently passing urine through her vagina. She has had treatment for an advanced cancer of the cervix 3 years earlier with radiotherapy and chemotherapy. All had gone well (cusp B) until a few weeks ago when the urinary problems had started. She had been examined in the clinic and unfortunately her tumor had returned and had created a hole between her bladder and vagina. Her kidneys are also failing so she is in cusp C, in other words she is no longer curable. She is unsuitable for surgery, further chemotherapy or radiotherapy. I told her these facts and that she had recurrent incurable cancer.

She said she had already guessed this and she was very angry. I then asked the vital question for **cusp C** which is: "I am very sorry to be giving you this news but is it that you are going to die in the next few weeks or months that is making you angry or is there something else which is troubling you?" It could be pain, constipation, etc. To this question the woman replied that she accepted the inevitability of impending death but, much worse, she had been told by someone else that nothing else could be done for her. I said, "I know that in terms of curing you, none of us can help you but what is your biggest problem right now?" To this she replied that her biggest problem now was her incontinence and the fact that she smelt of urine permanently. Because of this she could not go out, could not visit friends or be visited. I asked what other problems she was having to which she replied 'none'! At this point I was able to say to her that although I had no treatment myself, I had a colleague downstairs who is an interventional radiologist, a specialist in using x-rays to visualize the body, who could insert a tube into each kidney, to drain urine away, thus bypassing the hole in her bladder and rendering her dry and smell-free! (see Figure 3.6).

The patient went home the following day, and returned 2 months later in a terminal condition (**cusp D**). On return she said she had had a great 2 months, seen her friends, been to restaurants, pubs, etc. In this woman's case, death came within 24 hours and was peaceful. The fourth cusp lasts from hours to days and all interventions are only designed to ease the passing. Patients, in general, need no telling that this is where they have arrived although their

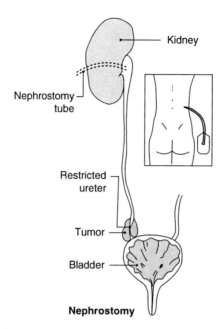

Figure 3.6. Nephrostomy

relatives may need help in arriving at this place. Care is focused on emotional support rather than medical intervention and, frequently, most of the patient's medicines can be stopped apart from pain relief. The death of a patient whose physical symptoms are well controlled and who is spiritually calm is an achievable goal to which all are entitled.

4. General Concepts of Surgical Management

The fact that you have bought this book is almost certainly because you have been diagnosed as having cancer. The process by which that diagnosis was made will, I know, have caused you great distress and seemed to have taken ages. For the majority of you, hopefully, it will have taken no more than a few weeks, but those few weeks will have been psychologically and/or physically painful and stressful. You will almost certainly have gone to your general practitioner, perhaps with a swelling in your tummy or some irregularity of bleeding, or perhaps with pain. Your general practitioner will have examined you, performed tests, and referred you either to a general gynaecologist or to some form of rapid assessment clinic, or perhaps directly to a gynecological cancer specialist. If you have attended the first two, then you may have been further referred to a gynecological cancer specialist. A gynecological cancer specialist will be a highly trained surgeon who will have specially trained in the area and will be somebody who you can feel certain is up to date in modern management of gynecological cancer, who understands the different types of treatment and will work within a large team of individuals. These teams meet at what are called multidisciplinary team meetings on a regular (weekly or fortnightly) basis. At these meetings, there are usually two or more surgeons, a radiotherapist, one or more medical oncologists who prescribe chemotherapy, a radiologist who takes and reads scans, x-rays, etc., a specialist oncology nurse, and a pathologist. All of these consultants may well have junior members in their respective teams, who will also attend these meetings and whom you may see during your care. These meetings ensure that you are offered the optimal treatment and that no one group, for example, the surgeon or the radiotherapist, can steer you into the wrong therapy.

What follows relates to referrals to the gynecologic oncologist when referrals are made for a cancer. This does not include patients with abnormal smears, who are sent for colposcopy. If you are in this category please go the section on colposcopy on page 43.

When you come to the clinic you will have your history taken; in other words, you will be asked about your medical "story" to date. This may be done by a medical student or a junior doctor in the first instance. Medical students take 5 years in training and your "junior doctor" in the UK may be qualified from 1 week to 12 years, i.e., some are not very "junior"! In the USA, the range is 1 week to 7 years. After the history you will be examined. This usually involves having both tummy and pelvic examinations. This should not be painful, but may occasionally be uncomfortable. Investigations are then ordered, including blood tests, usually for kidney function (urea and electrolytes), a full blood count to check for anemia, liver function tests, and a blood test called tumor markers. These tests tend to rise with cancers, although certain benign conditions can cause a rise as well. Scans and x-rays will be ordered for you. These may be by ultrasound, CT, MRI, or PET. None of these tests are painful. I can testify to this since I have had most of them! All these tests are designed to help determine whether the tumor is benign or cancerous/malignant. If there is a cancer, they will help to show if it has spread or not; this is called "staging." This will all be explained to you. Many people require to go on to have surgery and all the appropriate operations are described in the relevant chapter for each cancer type.

The general principle of how surgery works remains the same for all cancers. It is to remove an abnormal lump preferably with a 1 cm area of normal tissue around it (see Figure 4.1)

This is then analyzed in the pathology laboratory to determine whether it is cancerous and, if it is, has it been completely removed, thus avoiding the need for further treatment, while achieving a cure.

In summary, whenever one has surgery for a suspected cancer there are three outcomes: firstly, the problem proves to be benign and the surgery is likely to be the solution to the problem; secondly, it is cancerous but completely excised and the problem is solved; and thirdly, it is cancerous and perhaps not completely excised and further therapy will be required.

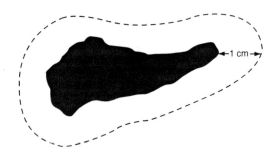

Figure 4.1. Tumor being removed with a minimum of a 1 cm clear margin around it

5. Sex, Cancer, and Surgery

When a woman develops cancer in her genital tract, be it the vulva (the outside of the vagina), the vagina itself, the cervix, uterus, tubes or ovaries, it is often the presumption that it is in some way related to sex. Often people harbor feelings of guilt as to whether they have done something wrong in the past that is now coming back to them in the form of a cancer. This impression has been further fostered by much of the tabloid press, where there regularly appear articles, suggesting that such and such a cancer is because of "promiscuity." The definition of "promiscuity," I always tell my students, is having had one more partner than your doctor! It is really a totally meaningless term. One person's promiscuity is another person's normality. Having said all of these, it is true that endometrial cancer is associated with never having been sexually active and not having had children. It is also true that taking the pill reduces your chances of ovarian cancer by 40%. It is also true that use of condoms protects one from bacterial sexually transmitted infections but not from virus infection, which is implicated in causing cervical cancer. Having said this, up to 85% of all men and women at some time in their lives will have human papilloma virus infection, irrespective of number of partners, but an incredibly low percentage of these will ever go on to develop cervical cancer itself. If you look in the cervical cancer chapter, you will see that there is much talk about cervical intraepithelial neoplasia (CIN), which is the cell change that takes place before women get cervical cancer. It has been, to my mind, extremely unfortunate that CIN, which should be stated by using the initials C, I, N has occasionally been referred to as "sin." It is obvious that anybody hearing a doctor talk about "sin" would immediately think that this must be related to something that they have done wrong! This is really just not the way it is!

Many women also worry as to what effect the treatment of their cancer will have upon sexual function. It is true to say that for the majority of gynecological cancers, you will be able to resume a normal sexual life afterwards.

Sex is a complicated mixture of the psychological and the physical. Whenever something goes wrong with the reproductive organs, this is likely to have some psychological effect at least in the first instance. Depending upon which part of the organs is affected this may affect sexual function afterwards, and in addition it obviously does depend upon the operation you have had as to what effect this may have. For this reason I have included a section on sexual aspects of treatments etc. in each of the chapters related to that particular cancer.

Overall, it is thought that in terms of orgasm there are four types of women: women who do not achieve orgasm, women who achieve orgasm through stimulation of the clitoris and external genitalia, women who achieve orgasm by deep penetration, and women who achieve orgasm by both routes. The famous "G" spot is a much disputed entity and if it exists, it perhaps exists in the cervix or related to the plexus of nerves in the front wall of the vagina, high up near the base of the bladder. These considerations are important, since for the majority of people having surgery for gynecological cancer this tends to involve either removal of an ovary or both ovaries, neither of which have any direct effect on sexual function, expect via hormones and the need for hormone replacement therapy (HRT). Removal of the uterus, again probably has no effect on sexual function. Removal of the cervix may affect deep orgasmic function, but probably does not in the majority of women. The evidence is that the majority of women following hysterectomy have an improved sex life and that removal of the cervix or not makes no difference to that pleasure. It is unusual for gynecological surgery to involve the vagina itself unless there is a tumor, which has spread onto the vagina.

Finally, for the small number of women where the vulva is affected, attempts, particularly in young women, are made to preserve as much vulval tissue as is possible, again with a view to preserving sexual function. Even women who have had a vulvectomy may still be capable of achieving orgasm, via the deep vaginal stimulation route. There is no doubting that radiotherapy to the pelvis greatly reduces the elasticity of pelvic organs and this can have a deleterious effect on sex. In addition, it can be associated with dryness although there are good vaginal lubricants available to alleviate dryness. It is extremely important that if you are having sexual problems you bring this up with your gynecological oncologist or with the specialist nurse, since there are usually things that can be done to help matters. There is a natural reticence on the part of many doctors/ nurses to directly ask about this area and a natural reticence on the part of the patients to not ask either.

Specific Cancers

6. Cervical Cancer and Precancer (Cervical Intraepithelial Neoplasia)

General Facts

No one knows exactly how common cervical cancer is. The "incidence" or rate varies in different parts of the world and in different parts of each country. The disease is more common in cities and less common in rural areas. It tends to be commoner in populations with lower socioeconomic status although higher economic status is no bar to developing the disease.

Cervical cancer is known to be associated with smoking because smoking has a direct effect on local immune cells in the cervix. It is also known to be associated with a poor immune system, for example, after having had an organ transplant and needing immunosuppressive drug treatment or as a result of human immunodeficiency virus (HIV) infection. It is very important to say that the vast majority of women who have cervical intraepithelial neoplasia (CIN) do not have HIV or, for that matter, have had an organ transplant. In addition, women with an abnormal smear should not think that they are at increased risk of having HIV.

Most women when they have an abnormal smear test believe that they have cervical cancer. This is almost always untrue. Long before developing cervical cancer, cell changes take place in the cervix and these are graded into CIN 1, 2, and 3. CIN stands for cervical intraepithelial neoplasia, i.e., NOT cancer but PRE-cancer. Cancers can spread but CIN cannot. Even before development of CIN 1, smears become borderline first. As can be seen from the diagram, you can draw arrows showing that some women's smears go from normal to borderline and then from borderline to CIN 1, progressing to CIN 2 and finally to CIN 3 (see Figure 6.1). If you had a CIN 3 diagnosis (and had no treatment) and did nothing about it, you would have a 30% chance that by the time 20 years had gone by you would have developed cervical cancer. Conversely, you would have a 20% chance that your smear would have gone back to normal on its own and a 50% chance that the smear would still remain as CIN 3. CIN 1, 2, and 3 cause no symptoms; they cause no pain, no bleeding, and no discharge, and in fact in themselves are not a problem. The problem is that they may develop into cervical cancer if left untreated. The lesser condition of CIN 1 has a higher chance of returning to normal with an approximately 50% chance of returning to normal within 6–12 months of diagnosis. This is the reason why you may have been told that you have an abnormal smear but the only action being taken is to repeat the smear a few months later. This particularly applies to borderline smears, again where there is a good chance of resolution (50–60%) happening without you requiring any treatment at all. The factors which primarily make some women's smears go from normal through to CIN 3 and others not, tend to be either heavy smoking or, more commonly, the acquisition of a type of virus called HPV, which stands for human papilloma virus. There are many types of HPV, some of which cause warts on the genitals (HPV 6 + 11) and others on the fingers. The types of HPV which cause CIN (HPV 16, 18, 31, 33, 35, 39, 45, 51, 52, 56, 58, 59, and 68) do not, however, cause warts. This can often lead to confusion since colloquially HPV is often known as "wart virus," confusion being that the types of HPV that cause CIN do **not** cause warts.

To create further difficulties in this part of the explanation, when you have a standard smear test taken there may be cells seen, which are 'suggestive of HPV'. This does not mean that you actually have HPV and it is not possible from looking at these cells to see which type of HPV is present, or even if it is HPV and not some other virus. Epstein Barr virus, which causes glandular fever, can cause this type of cell change but does **not** cause CIN. The only way to do this is by direct test for the virus. This direct test is not available in many clinics. Where the test is available there may be two tests: DNA and mRNA. If mRNA is positive, then it is likely that progression will take place unless there is treatment and therefore treatment will usually be offered. If the DNA is positive but the mRNA negative it is likely that things will return to normal without

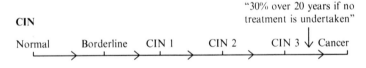

Figure 6.1. Sliding scale from normal to cervical cancer

Table 6.1. Action in the event of cervical smear result

Result	Action
Normal	Repeat as per national policy
Inflammatory/borderline (in the USA = ASCUS)	Screen for STIs, repeat at 6 months, utilize HPV testing
Suggestive of CIN 1 (in the USA = ASCUS)	? Colposcopy, repeat at 6 months, utilize HPV testing
Suggestive of CIN 2 (in the USA = HSIL	Refer for colposcopy
Suggestive of CIN 3 (in the USA = HSIL)	Refer for colposcopy
Suggestive of invasion (cancer) (v. unusual result)	Refer for colposcopy, urgent

treatment. In clinics where DNA testing alone is available persistence of a positive DNA test will lead to treatment.

For those clinics, which have access to the HPV testing kit, the results are used as a method of determining whether to treat CIN 1 or not. CIN 2 and 3 are always treated and I will discuss the treatment shortly. CIN 1 is only treated if it is persistent and/or in the presence of a positive HPV test (if this test is available). If this test is not available then CIN 1 is only usually treated if it is present on two occasions at least 6 months apart. The actions taken, depending upon the result, are shown in Table 6.1.

Explanation As to How CIN Arises

The area of the cervix (neck of the womb) which has the potential to develop CIN is called the transformation zone and it is formed after puberty. Figure 6.2 shows what happens from puberty to menopause.

The inside of the cervix has fleshy cells called columnar cells and on the outside it has squamous cells. Squamous cells are tough cells. At puberty, under the influence of the hormones which are released in all women, the cervix undergoes a process of eversion (out turning). This means that the fleshy columnar cells appear out on the surface. The vagina is then colonized with bacteria; these bacteria are normal to have in the vagina. In fact not to have them is positively harmful; they are called lactobacilli. These lactobacilli are the same lactobacilli found in live yoghurt, which are often used to prevent thrush. They cause the acidity in the vagina to increase. This, however, causes the fleshy columnar cells to change their nature and become tougher and to change into the squamous cells (i.e., to transform). The area where this change has taken place is the area which has the capacity to develop CIN. This area is called the transformation zone and, as you can see from Figure 6.2, the transformation

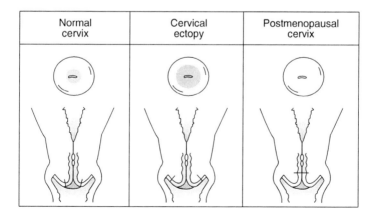

| Normal cervix | Cervical ectopy | Postmenopausal cervix |

Figure 6.2. Puberty to menopause: cervical changes

zone can vary from being on the outside of the cervix to the inside of the cervix. These are all just different variations of normal. They do, however, slightly alter the treatment depending on their position.

It is the fact that a precancerous condition exists in the cervix, in other words the cell change takes place many years before actual cancer, which makes it suitable for screening with smears. It is vitally important to realize that CIN (cervical intraepithelial neoplasia) is NOT cancer. Cancer means that a lesion has the capacity to metastasize, in other words to spread through the body. CIN has no such capacity. We also know that CIN 1 never directly becomes cervical cancer; it always becomes CIN 2–3 before becoming cervical cancer. It is these facts which make it safe to observe CIN 1 and make the relatively simple treatment offered for CIN 2 and 3 appropriate, giving a very high success rate in preventing women from developing cervical cancer.

One of the things, which often causes confusion is how often smears are undertaken and Table 6.2 shows the detection rates of CIN for cervical smears being taken at varying intervals. As you can see, the current National Health Service guideline is 3-yearly, which delivers a "hit rate" of 89%. Most other countries operate on the basis of an annual screening test, but this only gives a 4.5% gain in detection rate, while effectively doubling the cost of the entire program. It is also important to note that cervical cancer can be associated with low socioeconomic status and of course women in this category are less likely to go for smears, find out information about the subject or, for that matter, be reading a book like this. It is therefore, in terms of running a program effectively, most important to screen all of the people regularly rather than some of the people a lot!

There is an irony, since the smear program in the UK has had a lot of bad publicity over the last few years with regard to unreliability, and much unfavorable press when occasionally smears are missed. The irony is that the smear program is undoubtedly one of the "jewels in the crown" of the UK's NHS and in terms of the efficiency of the program's purpose, namely to reduce the incidence of invasive cancer within a specified population, it is one of the most successful programs in the world. Unfortunately, all medical tests have a false-positive and a false-negative rate, in other words they are reported as abnormal when there is no problem, or they are reported as normal when in fact there is a problem. It is for this reason that, over time, the more smears one has the better it is and the more accurate it is. The long time that CIN takes to develop into invasive cancer also makes it a very suitable thing for screening purposes. The false-negative rate of smears, namely when they are reported as normal

Table 6.2. Detection rates for cervical screening* at varying screening intervals (%)

10-yearly	64
5-yearly	84
3-yearly	89
Annualy	93.5

*Sexually active women are screened between the ages of 20 and 69 years

when in fact they are abnormal, is down to laboratory error or down to error in taking the smear. It is possible to take the smear from not quite the right area, although this happens rarely.

The Way the Smear Is Taken

You may notice when you go to the doctor that they vary in how they take your smear and this is dependent upon the position of the transformation zone; in other words, the area on the cervix which has the capacity to become abnormal varies from woman to woman and within the same woman over her lifetime. Sometimes it is possible to just use the spatula. Sometimes one should use the spatula at both ends and sometimes a spatula and a brush. The sample is then put on a slide and sent to a laboratory for reading. In addition, in some clinics, what is called liquid cytology (a Thin prep smear®) is used, which utilizes a device called the "broom." This device has the advantage that one can also directly test for human papilloma virus from the same sample and run a screen for other infections.

When you have a smear test it is either reported as normal or abnormal and the standard approach has already been shown in Table 6.1. In the event of an inflammatory smear, a screen for infection is undertaken. This tests routinely for Chlamydia, gonorrhea, Group B streptococcus, trichomonas, candida, and bacterial vaginosis. It is important to say that the Group B streptococcus and bacterial vaginosis are not sexually transmitted. Candida can be, but you can have candida and be a nun! Chlamydia is a sexually transmitted agent, but is not a venereal disease, i.e., discovery of it does not mean that you or your partner has been unfaithful to each other. The same does not apply to gonorrhea, which is a statutory venereal disease; in other words, it is suggestive of either you or your partner having had another partner. Having said this, there are certain tests for gonorrhea, which are used for rapid testing and these can be positive when you do not actually have gonorrhea. This is called a false-positive and occurs because of a cross-reaction of the test with a nonsexually transmitted throat bacteria. It is important to point out that human papilloma virus is extremely common. Approximately 85% of all men and women will have human papilloma virus at some point in their lives and while it is a marker of sexual activity, it is in no way a venereal disease. In fact if >50% of the population has something, then it cannot be regarded as abnormal to have it – more like it is normal to have it. Of the 85% who have HPV, the vast majority do not ever get a problem from it, only 5–10% getting an abnormal smear. We do not treat the male partner or the woman for HPV unless it is the variety which causes warts. These are treated because of their unsightly nature. Also remember that the type of HPV which causes warts (HPV 6 + 11) does not cause CIN. Most women with HPV will clear it themselves within an 18-month period. One exception to this may be women who smoke heavily because of smoking's effect on the immune cells, which inhibits the ability to naturally clear the virus. If you have an abnormal smear, you will be sent for a colposcopy.

Colposcopy

This word is derived from *colpos*, which is the Greek for vagina, and "scopy,"
to look. And in the same way as your doctor or practice nurse took the smear
by looking at your cervix with the naked eye, the only difference is that a

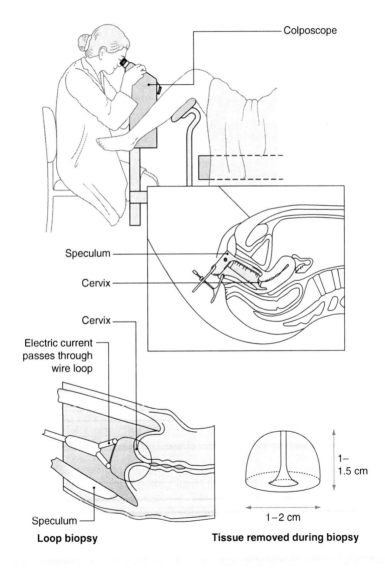

Loop biopsy

Tissue removed during biopsy

colposcopist, i.e., a gynecologist performing the colposcopy, will look at your cervix through the same type of speculum (viewing instrument), but this time looking down a binocular microscope (see Figure 6.2). This is not a painful examination, but the binocular microscope allows a 4–20 times normal magnification. When you go to the colposcopy clinic you can expect the gynecologist to take a history from you and then to explain to you that they will probably repeat your smear. They will explain that smears are designed to detect precancer and not cancer. Assuming that your doctor/nurse who originally took your smear has thought that your cervix looked normal, the chances of you having a cancer are incredibly low. Cancers are almost always seen by directly looking at the cervix and there is no requirement for a colposcope/microscope. CIN is a microscopic condition; in other words, it is not visible with the naked eye, but only with a microscope. The doctor will then give you a similar explanation to the one given in the previous pages with respect to CIN. You will then be taken through to another room where you will be placed on a couch (Figure 6.2) and the examination will be undertaken. Dyes are placed on the cervix. The first dye is usually merely saline (salt water), which is designed to clean the cervix. This will then be followed by a very dilute solution of acetic acid (vinegar). This does not cause stinging or pain. The final dye placed may be iodine (unless you are allergic to it). Occasionally, this can cause slight discomfort. If it does, washing with saline (salt water) gives immediate relief. Depending on what is seen, biopsies (small samples) may be taken from the cervix. The doctor may suggest that you cough, which makes the cervix bounce down and makes it easier to get the sample. It also usually has the advantage that you do not feel the sample being taken at all, which nobody believes until after they have had the sample taken. Occasionally, a slight "nip" is felt at the time of sampling. This sample will then be sent for analysis along with the repeat smear test and the colposcopic findings to allow a judgment to be made. Some clinics operate a

----

Figure 6.3. Colposcopy and treatment of abnormal smear

- Colposcopy is carried out if the smear test shows up abnormalities in the cervical cells. A colposcope is a microscope that magnifies the cervix.
- Colposcopy is a painless, outpatient procedure. You will be asked to lie on your back with your legs in supports.
- A plastic or metal instrument called a speculum is inserted into the vagina to hold the walls of the vagina apart. The speculum is similar to that used for a smear.
- Dilute acetic acid, and possibly iodine, will be painted onto your cervix to show up any abnormalities. Small samples of tissue, called biopsies, may be taken from the cervix and sent to the laboratory for analysis. These procedures do not hurt, but may be a bit uncomfortable.
- During colposcopy, abnormal cervical cells can be removed or destroyed in a number of ways. The most common is called loop biopsy or LLETZ. A local anesthetic is injected to numb your cervix. This is not painful, but may be uncomfortable. A small piece of tissue containing the abnormal cells is then removed using an electrical current; the sample removed is about the size of a marble. Other methods involve heating or freezing the area with the abnormal cells, or removing or destroying it using a laser.
- You are likely to have discharge and abnormal bleeding for a few weeks after treatment. If the bleeding is heavy or if the discharge becomes offensive, consult your doctor.

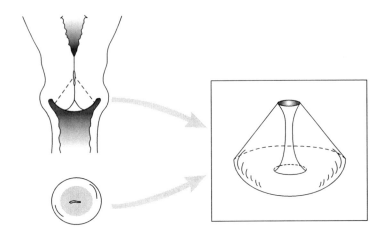

Figure 6.4. Local treatment of the transformation zone

policy of "see and treat," whereby if there is a lesion seen, treatment is undertaken then and there, which is described below. Certainly for appearances on the cervix that suggest CIN 1, very few people would do "see and treat," and for the appearances of CIN 2 and 3, many people are prepared to take a biopsy and wait for confirmation before proceeding onto treatment at a later date. The advantage of having "see and treat" is that it saves time and everything is dealt with in one go. The disadvantage is that there are usually high anxiety levels at the first visit to the clinic and it may be easier to get "used" to the colposcopy before moving onto the treatment.

Treatment of Abnormalities

It used to be, in the past (up until 15–20 years ago), that the treatments had to be dealt with as an inpatient, under general anesthetic. These were done using a knife to remove an area from the cervix (see Figure 6.3). Over the last 15–20 years a number of treatments have become available for outpatient use. The first of these was freezing therapy (cryotherapy) and this is still sometimes used for treatment of CIN 1. In persistently borderline smears it has about an 80% chance of working, is simple to use and pain-free, except for slight period like cramping pain occasionally. It does not require any local anesthetic.

The next treatment that became available was laser treatment. Most people have now moved away from using laser treatment partly because it takes quite some time to undertake the treatment, particularly if one wishes to produce a sample to send to the Pathology Department. Most clinics now use a large loop excision of the transformation zone (LLETZ) (Figure 6.2). Needle excision of the transformation zone (NETZ) can also be undertaken. Both of these allow removal of an ellipse of tissue as shown in the diagram, which allows both removal of the abnormal area and further investigation of the abnormal area, all effectively in one episode. In a further small number of people who have precancerous change on the vagina (VAIN) the laser is still used.

A very small number of women will be found, either on examination by their GP or on examination in the colposcopy clinic, to have a cervical cancer (cervical carcinoma). This is a different phenomenon from CIN. As stated earlier, CIN is the microscopic change which precedes cancer, usually by many years. Usually a person with cervical cancer is referred to the colposcopy clinic because the doctor taking the smear recognizes that the cervix has appeared very abnormal and makes an immediate referral. Occasionally, the referral may be because the smear is suggestive of malignancy. Occasionally, the LLETZ loop sample may show a cancer which was previously unsuspected. This is very uncommon. The other method by which women sometimes come to see the gynecologist is because they have had problems, e.g., bleeding between periods or bleeding after sex, and are seen and the doctor or nurse recognizes a cancer. With an effective screening program this has become a much rarer way of people being diagnosed.

Cervical Cancer

Whenever a cancer is diagnosed it is "staged." This refers to whether it has spread or not. When a cancer is "named" it is always "named" after where it has started, e.g., lung cancer has arisen in the lung. Sometimes it is not clear where the cancer has started; this is called an "unknown primary." Thus, cancer in the cervix starts in the cervix and can, as it spreads, move slowly through the cervix and onto the vagina or out to the side of the cervix. In addition, it can also spread into the lymph nodes. Occasionally, it can spread further toward the bladder or bowel. It very rarely spreads through the bloodstream, and therefore it is a type of cancer that has a relatively high cure rate and the cure is usually obtained by therapies which concentrate on the pelvic area. The first investigations once a diagnosis of cancer is suspected are to determine whether the cancer has spread or not. These incorporate blood tests, chest x-ray, and some form of scanning of the pelvis and the lymph nodes within the pelvis. It usually involves you being taken to theater for a "staging procedure." This is not in any way a curative procedure, but is designed to determine where the tumour is. This usually encompasses looking in the bladder (cystoscopy), looking in the vagina (colposcopy), looking in the rectum/colon (sigmoidoscopy), coupled up with the scan (see Figure 6.5). Staging is shown in Table 6.3.

All staging refers to the FIGO classification, which stands for Federation Internationale Gynaecologie Oncologie; this is an international committee which has agreed the exact classification of each cancer in gynecology. This is very important so that different hospitals, countries, etc. can compare their results for each cancer stage by stage. You can imagine that if somebody has a new idea for treating a type of cancer it is very important to know which stages it is suitable for and to assess if it works.

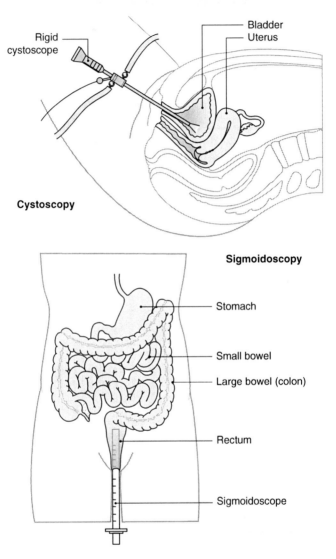

Figure 6.5. Cystoscopy, biopsy, and sigmoidoscopy

- Treatment of cervical cancer depends on the stage that the disease has reached. This is a measure of the size of the tumor and how far it has spread. Your doctor may carry out several different investigations (including a thorough pelvic examination), often under general anesthetic.

- A piece of tissue, called a biopsy, may be removed in the colposcopy clinic or while you are anesthetized. This is then sent to the laboratory for analysis.

Table 6.3. FIGO staging of cervical cancer

Stage 0	Intraepithelial neoplasia CIN 1, CIN 2, CIN 3.
Stage I	The carcinoma is strictly confined to the cervix, extension to the uterine corpus should be disregarded.
Ia	Preclinical carcinomas of the cervix (i.e., those diagnosed by microscopy only). All gross lesions even with superficial invasion are stage 1b. Invasion is limited to measured stromal invasion with a maximum depth of 5 mm and no wider than 7 mm. Measurement of the depth of invasion should be from the base of the epithelium, either surface or glandular, from which it originates. Vascular space involvement, either venous or lymphatic, should not alter the staging.
Ia1	Minimal microscopically evident stromal invasion. The stromal invasion is no more than 3 mm deep and no more than 7 mm in diameter.
Ia2	Lesions detected microscopically that can be measured. The measured invasion of the stroma is deeper than 3 mm but no greater than 5 mm, and the diameter is no wider than 7 mm.
Ib	Clinical lesions confined to the cervix, or preclinical lesions greater than stage 1a.
Ib1	Clinical lesions less than 4 cm in size.
Ib2	Clinical lesions greater than 4 cm in size.
Stage II	Involvement of the vagina except the lower third, or infiltration of the parametrium. No involvement of the pelvic sidewall.
IIa	Involvement of the upper two-thirds of the vagina, but not out to the sidewall.
IIb	Involvement of the parametrium, but not out to the sidewall.
Stage III	Involvement of the lower third of the vagina. Extension to the pelvic sidewall. On rectal examination there is no cancer-free space between the tumour and the pelvic sidewall. All cases with a hydronephrosis or non-functioning kidney should be included, unless this is known to be attributable to another cause.
IIIa	Involvement of the lower third of the vagina, but not out to the pelvic sidewall if the parametrium is involved.
IIIb	Extension onto the pelvic sidewall and/or hydronephrosis or nonfunctional kidney.
Stage IV	Extension of the carcinoma beyond the reproductive tract.
IVa	Involvement of the mucosa of the bladder or rectum.
IVb	Distant metastasis or disease outside the true pelvis.

(continued)

Figure 6.5. (continued)

- Your bladder may be examined in a procedure called cystoscopy. A narrow telescope, called a cystoscope, is inserted into your urethra to examine the bladder for signs that it has been affected by the cancer. The urethra is the tube through which urine passes out of the body.
- The lower part of the bowel may be examined in a procedure called sigmoidoscopy. A metal or plastic tube, called a sigmoidoscope, is inserted into the back passage.
- After these investigations, you may feel some discomfort when you go to the toilet, but this should pass within a day or so.
- Many patients with cervical cancer do not need these investigations.

Table 6.3. (continued)

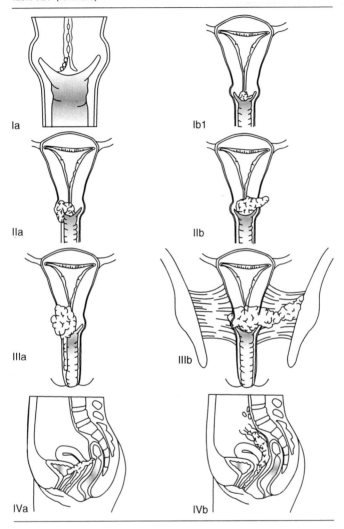

Ia

Ib1

IIa

IIb

IIIa

IIIb

IVa

IVb

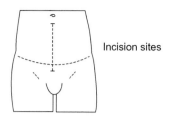

Incision sites

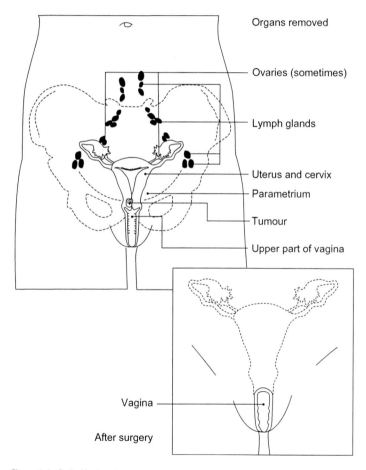

Organs removed

Ovaries (sometimes)

Lymph glands

Uterus and cervix

Parametrium

Tumour

Upper part of vagina

Vagina

After surgery

Figure 6.6. Radical hysterectomy

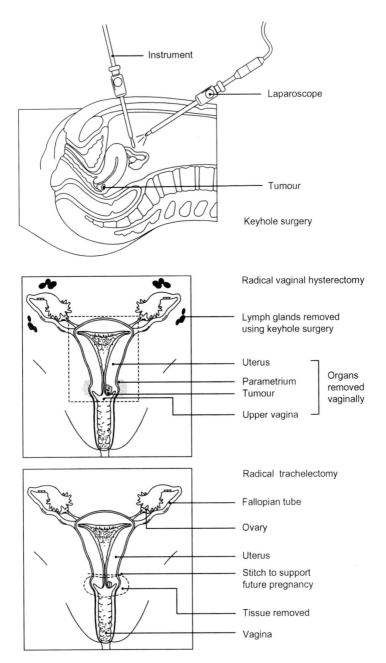

Instrument

Laparoscope

Tumour

Keyhole surgery

Radical vaginal hysterectomy

Lymph glands removed
using keyhole surgery

Uterus

Parametrium

Tumour

Upper vagina

Organs
removed
vaginally

Radical trachelectomy

Fallopian tube

Ovary

Uterus

Stitch to support
future pregnancy

Tissue removed

Vagina

Figure 6.7. Laparoscopically assisted radical vaginal hysterectomy and radical trachelectomy

The FIGO staging is reproduced here word for word and uses medical terminology. The medical terms are to be found in the glossary and also in the anatomy overview (pages 7–9). **This staging is not in any way related to the four cusps (A–D).**

The treatment offered to you after the staging procedure will depend upon the stage that your cancer is at. If your cancer is at stage 1A1, then treatment with a cone biopsy or simple hysterectomy, depending on whether you have completed your family or not, will be advised. The cure rate here is virtually 100%. Please see the earlier in the chapter for a more in-depth description of a cone biopsy.

Stage IA2 Cancer

The treatment of this type of cancer is highly specific to each patient. For some, treatment by cone biopsy alone may be the correct thing to do. For others a radical hysterectomy may be the correct thing, and for those wishing to retain fertility, a procedure called radical trachelectomy may be the appropriate operation. These operations are described separately at the end of the chapter (see Figure 6.6).

Stage IB1 Cancer

These cancers are usually managed by either radical hysterectomy or a radical trachelectomy depending on whether you have completed your family. Radical hysterectomy does not necessarily entail removal of your ovaries, and this is a separate issue, again depending upon your age. For those wishing fertility sparing surgery in the form of trachelectomy if your tumor is less than 2cms in diameter you are more likely to be offered the vaginal procedure. If the tumor is more than 2cms the abdominal procedure is preferable (see Figure 6.7).

Stage IB2 Cancer

These cancers are usually managed by radiotherapy and chemotherapy and unfortunately they are not normally regarded as safe options for preserving fertility. Radiotherapy and chemotherapy are described in Chapter 12.

Stage IIA–IV Cancer

Stage IIA, IIB, IIIA, IIIB, and IV are all also treated with chemotherapy and radiotherapy as described in Chapter 12.

7. Ovarian Cancer (Including Cancer of the Fallopian Tube)

This chapter is almost exclusively written around the subject of ovarian cancer, not fallopian tube cancer. Fallopian tube cancer is a very rare condition and when it does arise, it follows a very similar course to that of ovarian cancer. It is "staged" in the same way and it is treated in the same way and the staging refers to how far the cancer has spread. Because of the great similarities, no further mention will be made of fallopian tube cancer in this chapter, but what is written here relates to ovarian cancer, which would apply to fallopian tube cancer as well.

General Facts

Of all the cancers affecting women, lymphoma, cancer of the breast, colon, and uterus are more common than cancer of the ovary. Cancer of the ovary accounts for approximately one quarter of all gynecological cancers. Overall the risk for women is approximately 1:70 of developing this type of tumor. It tends to occur most commonly between the ages of 55 and 59, but can occur at any age. It tends to be commoner in white women than in black women. There has been an increasing incidence of this cancer over the last 40 years, which may be accounted for by women having smaller families, increased affluence, and an increasingly high fat diet. A number of factors are associated with ovarian cancer and these include never being pregnant, infertility, high fat diet, higher socioeconomic status, family history, celibacy, early menopause, and exposure to talcs and asbestos. Ovarian cancer is also associated with breast and endometrial cancer and all three of these cancers are associated with high fat diet. There is possibly an association with ovarian stimulatory drugs, but there is certainly no evidence of an association between in vitro fertilization (IVF) and ovarian cancer unless there have been multiple cycles. As might be expected, factors which suppress egg production, namely the oral contraceptive pill, and multiple pregnancies are protective against ovarian cancer. **The oral contraceptive pill if taken for 5 years continuously gives a 40% reduction in the risk of ovarian cancer.**

Screening

Much effort is currently being made to develop a screening test for ovarian cancer. Screening programs for cancer are ideal if they identify a change within an organ before cancer itself develops, and this change is easily treated and, for that matter, easily detected. For this reason, screening for cancer of the cervix is ideal because there is a precancerous phase, which takes up to two to three decades to develop into cancer and is easily detected by taking a smear. In contrast, the mammogram program for breast cancer is not designed to detect a precancerous phase, but rather to detect early cancer, the theory being that if you detect the cancer early you are more likely to cure it than if you detect it late. Both the breast and the cervix have the advantage of being easily accessible. The breast can be mammogrammed and the cervix can be smeared. One of the great difficulties with the ovary is that it is an internal organ and it is difficult to detect changes within it by examination alone. Also, to further complicate matters, the ovary is a naturally "cystic" structure; it normally forms a cyst every month when it produces an egg, which is exactly what it is designed to do. If you scan women, most of them will have small ovarian cysts at one time or another and in fact every month in a woman who is fertile, follicles will be developing and will show as cysts on scans. After the eggs have been produced a little cyst called the corpus luteum, which produces progesterone, the natural hormone to support pregnancy, will also be seen. This obviously means that if you utilize scanning to screen people for ovarian cysts, a very high number of the scans will show positive, whereas virtually none of these women will in fact have cancer.

A number of ways of screening for ovarian cancer have been investigated, including performing vaginal examination and ultrasound scans, and measuring a blood test called Ca-125. Ca-125 is a protein which can be produced by ovarian cancer. It is, however, also produced in benign gynecological conditions such as endometriosis and fibroids, which further complicates matters. A new area of development is called proteomics, which is looking at detecting various proteins in the bloodstream that may be produced early on in the development of ovarian cancer.

Currently, if you are to be screened for ovarian cancer, this will encompass having ultrasound scans performed with the probe within the vagina (transvaginal ultrasound), coupled with measurements from blood tests of Ca-125 and with vaginal examinations. Even combining these tests together carries a high false-positive rate. This means that it is much more likely you will be told that you might have a cancer when in fact you do not, and you would have to undergo surgical investigation to determine whether you do or you do not have a cancer. At the moment, because of this high risk of subjecting women who have no problem to unnecessary surgery, screening is limited within the National Health Service in the UK to patients who have two close relatives (mother or sister) who have had ovarian cancer. In North America and the remainder of Western Europe and in private practice within the UK, having one close relative with ovarian cancer is usually seen as being adequate to commence screening, although statistically gynecologists may be placing their patients at increased risk and anxiety because of the high rate of overdiagnosis of the problem. In the main, ovarian cancer, if it is detected, is detected in its true cancerous form, rather than in a precancerous form. In other words, it is a bit like breast cancer where you aim to detect the cancer earlier rather than later and thus increase the cure rate. There is, however, an intermediate form for problems in the ovary called "borderline." We believe that there is a "sliding scale" where normal can go to borderline, which can then go onto ovarian cancer, and this is shown in Figure 7.1.

"Borderline" is not a true cancerous state; in other words, it does not have the ability to spread, other than directly but not through the blood stream or through the lymph system.

Where patients have actually developed a cancer, this is "staged." Staging refers to how far the tumor has spread and Table 7.1 shows a representation of this.

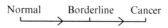

Figure 7.1. Sliding scale normal to cancer

Table 7.1. FIGO staging of ovarian cancer

Stage I	Growth limited to the ovaries
Ia	Growth limited to one ovary, no ascites
	No tumor on the external surface, capsule intact
Ib	Growth limited to both ovaries, no ascites
	No tumor on the external surface, capsule intact
Ic	Tumor either stage 1a or b but with tumor on the surface of one or both ovaries on with capsule ruptured or with ascites present containing malignant cells or with positive peritoneal washings
Stage II	Growth involving one or both ovaries with pelvic extension
IIa	Extension and/or metastases to the uterus and/or tubes
IIb	Extension to other pelvic tissues
IIc	Tumor either Stage IIa or b, but with ascites or positive peritoneal washings
Stage III	Growth involving one or both ovaries with intraperitoneal metastases outside the pelvis and/or positive retroperitoneal or inguinal nodes, or tumor limited to the true pelvis with histologically proven malignant extension to small bowel or omentum, superficial liver metastases equals Stage III.
IIIa	Tumor grossly limited to the true pelvis with negative nodes but with histologically confirmed microscopic seeding of abdominal peritoneal surfaces.
IIIb	Tumor of one or both ovaries, histologically confirmed implants of abdominal peritoneal surfaces, none exceeding 2 cm in diameter, nodes negative.
IIIc	Abdominal implants 2 cm in diameter and/or positive retroperitoneal nodes or inguinal nodes.
Stage IV	Growth involving one or both ovaries with distant metastases. If pleural effusion is present, there must be positive cytology to allot a patient to stage IV. Parenchymal liver metastases equal stage IV.

(continued)

Table 7.1. (continued)

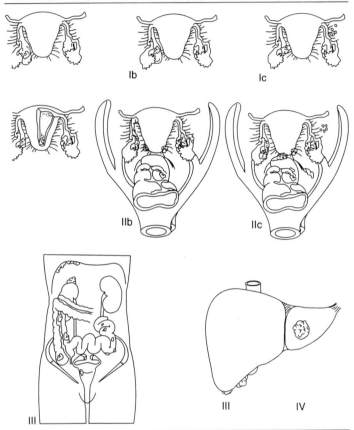

All staging refers to the FIGO classification, which stands for Federation Internationale Gynaecologie Oncologie; this is an international committee who have agreed the exact classification of each cancer in gynecology. This is very important so that different hospitals, countries, etc. can compare their results for each stage. You can imagine that if somebody has a new idea for treating a type of cancer it is very important to know which stage it is suitable for and to assess if it works. The FIGO staging is reproduced word for word and has highly technical terms. These are explained in the glossary (page 123) and in the anatomy overview (pages 7–9). **This staging (I–IV) is NOT in any way related to the Cusps (A–D).**

This staging of ovarian cancer is determined by the results of the operation which you may be about to undergo, or have undergone.

Diagnosis

There are various routes by which you may have come to your gynecological cancer specialist. This may be because you have felt a lump in your tummy, or on examination a lump in your tummy has been found. It may also be that you have had a scan for one reason or another, which has detected a cyst on the ovary. Whichever of these applies to you, when you arrive at the gynecological cancer clinic, you will meet your gynecological cancer specialist who will talk you through the possibilities. He/she will wish to do blood tests. These will include tests for anemia, tests of your blood salts, (kidney function), the function of your liver and your tumor markers. Tumor markers are blood tests which detect proteins produced by cancers and in general people will check for Ca-125, which can go up with ovarian cancer, and also another marker called carcinoembryonic antigen (CEA). This tends to be raised with bowel cancer. In addition, a Ca 19-9 may be checked which rises with ovarian, bowel and pancreatic cancer. The specialist will perform an examination of your tummy and pelvis and perhaps take a cervical smear, if you have not had this done recently. They will then order a computed tomography (CT) scan or possibly a magnetic resonance imaging (MRI) scan to further determine how things are in your pelvis and abdomen. If you have not had an ultrasound scan, they will arrange this too.

In general, we utilize a formula called the "risk of malignancy index" (RMI). This is a way of determining whether women have a high chance that any cyst on their ovary is benign or whether it might be cancerous. If the risk of malignancy index is less than 200, this is regarded as a good result and if it is more than 200, then one has to tread more cautiously.

The risk of malignancy index encompasses a score which is related to your menopause. If you are before the menopause, then you score 1 and if you are after the menopause you score 3. It also relates to the findings on your ultrasound scan for which again you may score 1 or 3. Finally, it also relates to your Ca-125 level. To find your RMI we multiply your Ca-125 level, your ultrasound findings score, and your menopause status score. As you can imagine, if you are before the menopause and have a simple looking cyst, then you have to have a very high Ca-125 for there to be a problem. If you are after the menopause and have a complicated cyst, you would only need to have a relatively low Ca-125 to jump the threshold for the cyst requiring to be managed as if it were a cancer, even though it may well not be. This is illustrated in Table 7.2.

Table 7.2. Risk of malignancy index (<200 is reassuring, >200 requires further investigation)

Ca-125	X	Ultrasound findings	X	Menopause status
(0–36 = normal range)		(0 = no cyst 1 = cyst with one feature 3 = cyst with more than one feature)		(1 = not meno-pausal 3 = menopausal)

If you are somebody who has an RMI of less than 200, and if you are before the menopause, you may well be eligible for management by keyhole surgery. If, however, the RMI is over 200, it is still very possible that you do not have a cancer, but nobody can take a chance on this. An ovary with cancer cells in it can, under keyhole management, burst, and cancerous cells could then spread around the inside of your abdomen/tummy and spread the cancer. This would make a Stage Ia cancer, which is quite curable by surgery alone, into a Stage Ic cancer, which is still quite curable, but requires having chemotherapy as well as surgery.

Unfortunately, therefore, if your RMI is over 200, you have to be managed as if you may have a cancer. This means that you are required to be properly "staged" and the ovary that has the problem requires to be removed intact. This, therefore, almost always requires a midline opening of your tummy (midline laparotomy). This is shown in Figure 7.2.

If you are somebody who has a scan which is suspicious of a cancer that has spread outside the ovary, you will also require to have a midline opening of your tummy (midline laparotomy). This is designed to determine how much cancer is inside your abdomen and to remove as much of it as is possible.

There are four potential outcomes under this circumstance. One is that the tumor is completely removed so that there is no visible tumor left to the naked eye (complete macroscopic clearance of the tumor). The second is that the cancer is removed to the extent that there is no cancer left in your abdomen which is greater than 1 cm diameter in size; this is called an optimal debulk. The third is that a lot of cancer is removed, but there are still areas of tumor greater than 1–2 cm in size. The fourth is that the tumor is completely unremovable. The last eventuality that the tumor is not removable at all is extremely unlikely. Clearly, the first option is the best and the fourth option is the worst. The reason for

--→

Figure 7.2. TAH & BSO and omentectomy, and debulking surgery
- If your ovarian cancer is at an early stage, you will probably have a total abdominal hysterectomy and bilateral salpingo-oophorectomy (TAH & BSO). This involves removing the uterus, cervix, Fallopian tubes, and ovaries. The pelvic lymph glands may also be removed. The fat 'apron' in the abdomen (the omentum) is also removed in a procedure called omentectomy.
- The operation is carried out under general anesthetic. A catheter will drain urine from the bladder for a few days, and you will stay in hospital for about 1 week.
- Your doctor may not know whether your tumor is benign or cancerous or, if cancerous, how advanced it is, until the pathology report is available, usually 3–7 days after the operation.
- If the cancer is advanced, it is necessary to remove as much of the tumor as possible during the operation; this is called debulking surgery, and may involve bowel surgery. This does not cure ovarian cancer, but can delay or prevent complications such as bowel or kidney obstruction. It also makes chemotherapy, which is treatment with drugs that attack the cancer cells, more effective.
- If the cancer affects only one ovary, and you have yet to complete your family, a unilateral oophorectomy may be an option. This involves removing only the affected ovary. You may be recommended to have the other ovary removed with a hysterectomy later.

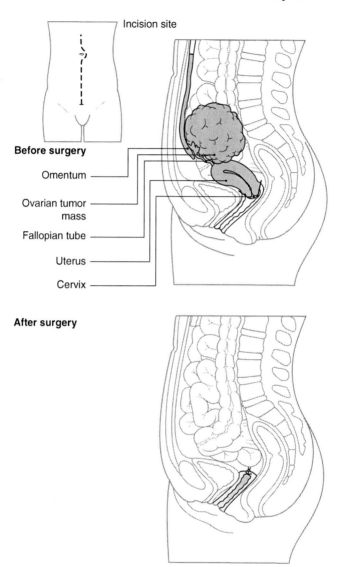

Incision site

Before surgery

Omentum

Ovarian tumor
mass

Fallopian tube

Uterus

Cervix

After surgery

this, apart from being self-evident, relates to how well chemotherapy will work for you. If there is only microscopic disease left the chemotherapy has a better chance of clearing it than if there are small lumps of cancer left. In turn, the chemotherapy is better at dealing with small lumps of tumor than large ones.

Surgery for Ovarian Cancer

Postmenopause/Family Completed

You will have a midline laparotomy, i.e., your tummy will be opened through a vertical incision (see Figure 7.2). You will have a hysterectomy, either total or subtotal, and this is explained elsewhere. You will have removal of the fallopian tubes and both ovaries. In addition the omentum, which is a fatty tissue that hangs from your stomach and transverse colon, will be removed. I have never met any patient who has ever heard of the omentum unless they were a doctor, nurse, or vet (see Figure 7.2). It is known as the "abdominal policeman" because it goes to where trouble is. Unfortunately, therefore, in the case of cancers, it goes to the cancer and picks up cancer cells, which is why it is an early place for the spread of cancer. It therefore requires to be removed. In other conditions, e.g., appendicitis, it goes to wall off the appendix. Prior to the surgical era (before 1900), the omentum could prove to be important if, for instance, one developed appendicitis. It is difficult to imagine that appendicitis, which is now such an easily treated condition, before 1900 and before surgery carried such a high chance of dying. The omentum did protect people at that time, although even with your omentum there was still approximately 25% chance of dying. Nowadays your omentum is something which you can certainly afford to lose. In addition, having removed the uterus, tubes, and omentum, many surgeons will have an analysis made of the tissues which are removed while you are still in the theater (frozen section). If there is a possibility that your cancer is confined to only one or both ovaries, they will then sample your lymph nodes along the main blood vessel, in the abdomen, the aorta, and from alongside the vessels in the pelvis. Your surgeon may also remove your appendix. All of these are designed to be absolutely certain as to how far the cancer has spread. The rationale behind this is that if you have a cancer that is confined to one ovary and it truly is confined to that ovary, then the only treatment that you need is surgery, which will confer a very high cure rate. If, however, the cancer has spread and if you do not take the right samples, you cannot know whether the cancer has spread or not, and then you would require to be treated with chemotherapy also.

For those women who have disseminated cancer, in other words it has spread outside the ovary, every effort will be made to remove (debulk) as much as possible. There is a very small chance that you may require to have some bowel removed and for this reason you will have had your bowel prepared before the operation with a drink/enema to empty it. This is designed to minimize the risk of colostomy where the bowel is diverted into a bag. Thankfully this is a rare occurrence.

Premenopause/Family not Completed

If you have not completed your family fertility-sparing surgery may be possible. This depends on what the preoperative investigations suggest. In addition, analyses can be undertaken during the operation (frozen section) to determine whether the tumor is benign, borderline, or cancerous, and if cancerous how far it has spread. Frozen section is fairly reliable but not 100%. In other words, occasionally the frozen section says there is no cancer and later it is discovered that there is. It is rarely the other way round, if the frozen section is positive for cancer it almost always is.

If your RMI lies below 200 all well and good it is highly unlikely that you have a cancer and fertility-sparing surgery is the order of the day possibly via a keyhole approach. If, however, it is above this, then you will require to be managed as if you have a cancer, even though you may not have one. Remember the best result at the end is that it is benign; this does not mean that you have had unnecessary surgery.

If the scans done preoperatively suggest that the tumor is confined to the ovary, you will be offered a midline laparotomy, removal of the affected ovary, and adjoining fallopian tube. This will then be analyzed during your operation (frozen section). While the pathologist is doing the analysis, the omentum is removed. If there are any other suspicious areas these will be biopsied. There are three possible results from the frozen section: benign, borderline, or cancer. If benign or borderline, the procedure will stop at this point. If it is cancer, then your surgeon will proceed to sample your para-aortic and pelvic lymph nodes and possibly biopsy the other ovary. Your appendix may also be removed. The procedure will then finish and you will have retained your organs of fertility. There is a very small chance that the full histology results which will be available 1 week later may necessitate further surgery, but this is very unlikely, and a chance many women believe worth taking.

If the preoperative scans suggest tumor in both ovaries they would both require frozen section and may both have to be removed. This still leaves the possibility of retaining the uterus, which would allow pregnancy with donated eggs at a future date. Unfortunately, if ovarian cancer is diagnosed it is not possible to store eggs/ovarian tissue since reimplantation at a future date may result in reimplanting the cancer as well as the eggs. Finally, if the scans suggest disseminated cancer, then assuming frozen section analysis is positive for cancer it will prove necessary to remove all the organs as in the operation described above for the postmenopausal woman. Thankfully, this is very uncommon but sadly removes all chance of child bearing.

Postoperative Care

Your surgeon will come and tell you what they've found within the first 24–48 hours after the operation. They will have much more data for you approximately 2–4 weeks later, when the results of all the samples have gone to the laboratory and been analyzed. It is only at this stage that the true stage, as shown on Page 53, of your cancer will be known.

If you have a Stage 1A cancer, which does not appear aggressive in terms of its type, then no further active treatment will be given to you and you will be followed up with regular hospital visits for the next 5–10 years.

This follow-up usually involves 3–4 monthly visits to the clinic with measurements of blood tests and examination of your abdomen/tummy and pelvis/vaginal examination and perhaps intermittent scans. It is very important to remember that one-off blood test results do not mean anything. It is trends that matter and this is demonstrated in the two diagrams opposite. One shows somebody who has blips up and down of their Ca-125 and the other shows someone whose Ca-125 continues to rise. Unfortunately for the person in the latter category, this means that they perhaps have a recurrence of their cancer, whereas blips up and down are not usually significant.

For the person with aggressive Stage 1a or Stage Ib or greater, where the cancer has spread out of the ovary, further management is always suggested and has been shown to be beneficial. This is usually with chemotherapy but occasionally can be with radiotherapy. Please refer to the chapter on chemotherapy and radiotherapy for more information on this if this applies to you. For the person who requires further management, the follow-up is again similar, with review every 3–4 months for the first 2 years, then every 6 months for the next 3 years, and then every year for the following 5 years. I would also suggest that if you have had or are going to have chemotherapy please refer to Chapter 3, since much of this chapter relates to people in this position.

8. Endometrial Cancer

General Facts

Cancer of the endometrium is the most common gynecological cancer and in fact the fourth most common cancer in women. It is one and a half times as common as ovarian cancer and three times as common as cervical cancer. It would appear that since the 1970s the number of women with endometrial cancer has risen, but commensurate with this rise has been a rise in the cure rate. This may be because of increasing awareness among women that when they have bleeding, particularly after their menstrual periods are finished, it is important that they attend their doctor for investigations. This has allowed earlier diagnosis of the condition and, as with all cancers, the usual rule is that the earlier you diagnose it, the higher is the cure rate. Most women tend to be diagnosed between the age of 50 and 60, but 20–25% will have a diagnosis made before the menopause and a small percentage (5%) will be diagnosed before the age of 40. This is why for those women who have menstrual upset, particularly when they are in their forties, investigation is always undertaken to make sure that they do not have endometrial cancer. The vast majority of people with menstrual upset do not have endometrial cancer, but unfortunately a small minority do. Even when women who are in the menopause start bleeding again, the majority of these women do not have endometrial cancer, although clearly investigation has to be done to make certain that this is not the diagnosis.

In terms of lifestyle issues which have effects on the development of endometrial cancer, the oral contraceptive pill and cigarette smoking appear to reduce the risk, while being overweight, never having been pregnant, and a late menopause all tend to increase the risk. In addition, the use of estrogen-only hormone replacement therapy (HRT) without any progesterone causes an increased risk. Nowadays, if you have a uterus all HRTs are prescribed with progesterone as well as estrogen. The progesterone may be given by tablets or via a Mirena coil. There is an association of endometrial cancer with diabetes mellitus. Tamoxifen therapy, which is given to women with breast cancer, also unfortunately increases the risk of endometrial cancer. It is most important to say that in terms of risks versus benefits, if one has had a breast cancer and is prescribed Tamoxifen therapy, the very small risk of getting endometrial cancer is very much outweighed by the reduced risk of getting one's breast cancer

Table 8.1. Sliding Scale from normal to endometrial cancer

Normal → Hyperplasia → Mild atypia → Moderate atypia → Severe atypia → Endometrial cancer	
No atypia	

back, and therefore it is vitally important to take the Tamoxifen therapy which has been prescribed.

Endometrial cancer happily carries a very high cure rate and while nobody would ever want to develop any form of cancer, there is no doubting that an endometrial cancer, which is detected early has close to 100% cure rate. Mercifully, many women are diagnosed early and hence the prognosis is excellent, with relatively simple therapy for the majority.

Many women believe that when they go for investigation for bleeding there are in essence two possibilities with respect to their diagnosis. One is that they have a benign condition and the other is that they have a cancerous condition. This is not the case with endometrial problems. There is effectively a sliding scale of abnormality which starts with normal and moves to hyperplasia; in other words, thickening of the endometrium. This thickening can have cells which are abnormal (the medical term being atypia) and which are graded mild, moderate, or severe. Finally, at the end of this sliding scale is endometrial cancer. This is shown in Table 8.1

In terms of treatment, simple thickening (hyperplasia) and hyperplasia with mild to moderate atypia can all be treated medically with progesterone therapy. Progesterone is a hormone that occurs naturally in women in the second half of their cycle, after they have produced an egg, and this drug can be used to stabilize the lining of the uterus, namely the endometrium. It can either be administered in tablet form or via the Mirena coil. For the more severe forms of atypia, surgical management in the form of hysterectomy is usually advocated since, for the woman with severe atypia, she has a 50% chance of developing an endometrial cancer if she is left untreated for 2 years. For the younger woman wishing to preserve her fertility other options may be possible, but are not without some element of risk and are discussed elsewhere (page 69).

How Is the Diagnosis Made?

For a woman who is past the menopause the development of bleeding will alert her to the fact that she should go to her doctor, and her doctor will refer her rapidly to a gynecologist for investigation of this bleeding. For a woman who is prior to the menopause, the usual method of being alerted is irregularity of her periods. Clearly, the majority of women coming up to the menopause tend to get some irregularity, which means that the vast majority of people who do get irregularity do not have cancer. It has to be said that the bleeding tends to be heavier and more frequent rather than less frequent in women who may have endometrial cancer. Most women going toward the menopause tend to have less frequent bleeding, rather than more frequent bleeding. A number of women are diagnosed as having endometrial cancer from their cervical smear. Although the cervical smear program is not in any way designed to detect endometrial cancer, it does sometimes pick up abnormal cells from the endometrium.

In the past when one arrived at the gynecologist, the investigation which was performed was dilatation and curettage (D&C). Dilatation refers to dilatation (opening) of the cervix and curettage refers to the process of scraping the inside of the uterus. This is no longer regarded as a proper investigation for endometrial cancer unless it is combined with the investigation of hysteroscopy. Hysteroscopy is where a small (3 mm wide) telescope is passed up through the cervix into the inside of the uterus, allowing visualization of the inside of the uterus. Hysteroscopy may be performed in the outpatient department under local anesthetic or, more commonly, in the operating theater, usually as a day-case procedure performed under general anesthetic. Practice, whether it is done as an inpatient or outpatient, varies from hospital to hospital. Certainly, if it proved impossible to insert the telescope in the outpatient department, then admission to the operating theater will be arranged on another day for the hysteroscopy under general anesthetic. When that is done, the cervix requires dilatation and once one has seen what is inside the uterus, curettage is effected to obtain a sample to send to the laboratory (see description at the end of the chapter).

The alternative to hysteroscopy and D&C is outpatient sampling using a pipelle sampler (see Figure 8.1). This allows cells to be sucked up from inside the uterus and sent to the laboratory for analysis. This is a "blind" procedure, where the doctor cannot see where the sample is being taken from, and for this reason an ultrasound scan is also performed. The ultrasound scan allows the doctor to assess the size of the uterus, the size of the ovaries, and the thickness of the endometrium. If the endometrium is thin (less than 4 mm), it is highly unlikely that an endometrial cancer is present. If the endometrial thickness is great (more than 12 mm), either postperiod or postmenopause, this is suspicious, and if there is nothing obtained on the outpatient sample, then you would be referred for a hysteroscopy to confirm that everything was all right. The trouble with outpatient sampling is that if no sample is obtained, and the bleeding continues or something is found on the sample, then the next investigation is to go for hysteroscopy and D&C (see Figure 8.2). For this reason many gynecologists will decide and advise you to go straight for the hysteroscopy and D&C, rather than doing outpatient sampling coupled with ultrasound. As can be seen from all that I have written above, there is quite a lot of variation as to how different doctors investigate. It suffices to say, though, that all are designed to maximize safety.

The scope of what may be detected is quite wide and in addition to what has been previously discussed, an alternative finding can be that of polyps. Polyps are fleshy growths which can arise in the endometrium or in the cervix. (They can also arise in your nose, throat, guts, etc.) The majority of polyps are benign, but having said this, some may have atypical changes as in Table 8.1, and very rarely they may prove to be cancerous.

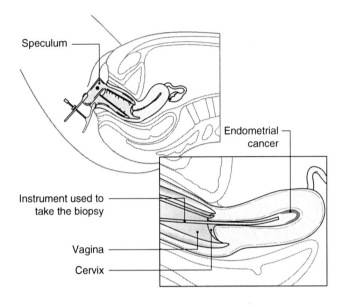

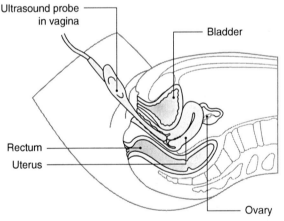

Figure 8.1. Endometrial biopsy and ultrasound

- Endometrial biopsy and ultrasound can both be used to investigate the cause of abnormal bleeding.
- An endometrial biopsy is a sample of tissue taken from the lining of the uterus, known as the endometrium. The biopsy is usually carried out as an outpatient procedure without an anesthetic.
- You will be asked to lie on your back with your legs apart. A plastic or metal instrument called a speculum is inserted into the vagina to hold the vaginal walls apart. A narrow plastic device is then passed into the vagina, through the cervix and into the uterus, where it is used to remove a piece of tissue. This is then sent to the laboratory.

What Happens Once the Diagnosis of Cancer Is Made

Having had the diagnosis of cancer made by your gynecologist, a number of investigations will then follow. You will have blood taken to check that you are not anemic, to check your blood salts (urea and electrolytes), and to check your liver function tests. You will almost certainly have an ECG to check your heart and you will have blood taken for cross-match so that if you bleed during potential treatment, blood is available for you. In addition, another kind of x-ray investigation, either computed tomography (CT) or magnetic resonance imaging (MRI) scanning, will take place.

All cancers are staged and the staging is called FIGO staging. FIGO (Federation Internationale Gynaecologique Oncologie) is an international committee who have agreed the exact classification of gynecological cancers. It is very important so that different hospitals, countries, etc. can compare their results for each cancer, stage for stage. You can imagine that if somebody has a new idea for treating a type of cancer it is extremely important to know which stage it is suitable for and to assess if it works. Table 8.2 shows the FIGO staging of endometrial cancer and alongside this are shown pictures which demonstrate each of the stages. The FIGO staging I–IV has NO relationship to the four cusps A–D.

Although the exact stage of your cancer can only be known after your surgery we try very hard with our preoperative investigations to get a good idea as to what stage your cancer is at before we take you to the operating theater. This allows us to tailor your treatment to the presumed stage you are at. However, the actual stage of your cancer is only known after you have had surgery. The mainstay of surgical treatment is an operation called total abdominal hysterectomy and bilateral salpingo-oophorectomy. This means removal of your uterus, cervix, fallopian tubes, and ovaries. This operation is shown pictorially in Figure 8.3, along with advice as to recovery etc. Some surgeons perform this procedure laparoscopically, as shown in Figure 8.3

There are debates among gynecologists as to whether other things should be removed at the same time as the uterus, tubes, and ovaries. This partly depends upon the estimate of the stage of your cancer from the scans and blood tests which have been performed, and also may partly depend upon the center at which you are being managed. There is agreement that for the earliest cancers, Stage IA, a simple hysterectomy and removal of tubes and ovaries alone is adequate treatment. For cancers which have spread into the muscle of

---

Figure 8.1. (continued)

- Endometrial biopsy is not usually painful. If you have not been pregnant, however, your cervix might be tightly closed. If this is the case, local anesthetic can be used to numb the cervix, and a metal instrument can be used to open it gently. Sometimes a general anesthetic is needed.
- You can get back to normal straight away after an endometrial biopsy, but you may have spotting of blood for a few days afterwards. Laboratory results should be with your doctor in about a week.
- With ultrasound, a probe is gently placed in the vagina, and the image of the uterus is seen on a screen. Scan results are available immediately, but you may have to wait for your doctor to interpret them and inform you.

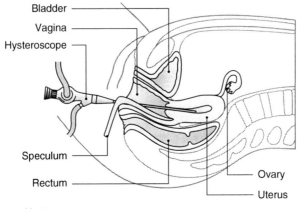

Hysteroscopy

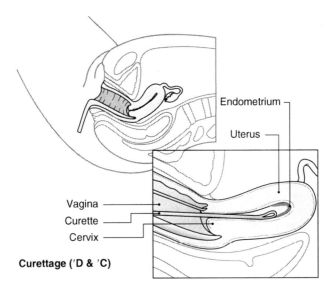

Curettage ('D & 'C)

Figure 8.2. Hysteroscopy and curettage

- Hysteroscopy is a method of examining the uterus using a small telescope called a hystero-scope. It may be carried out under local anesthetic in the outpatient clinic, or as a day-case procedure under general anesthetic. It takes about 20 minutes.

- If you are awake, you will be asked to lie on your back with your legs in supports. The hystero-scope is passed though the vagina and cervix into the uterus. Gas or liquid is used to distend the uterus slightly to make the examination easier.

the uterus or elsewhere, there is debate as to whether it is valuable to remove the lymph glands at the same time as removing the uterus. Removal of the lymph glands is shown in Figure 8.3. In addition, some surgeons believe that it is better to just sample the lymph nodes so that if they are found to be positive, then you would be referred for further treatment. Other surgeons go for a more aggressive approach and actually remove all of the lymph nodes in the hope that this may improve the cure rate.

As you can imagine, the fact that there are several different approaches means that nobody in truth actually knows the right answer as to what should be done, and for this reason there are a number of studies currently running within the UK and in the USA to try and answer these questions.

In addition to removal of the lymph nodes, some surgeons advocate removal of the omentum, which most people have not heard of, but is a fatty structure which hangs from the stomach and transverse colon and is also called the "abdominal policeman." It gets this nickname because it goes to where the trouble is. Unfortunately, if one has a cancer the omentum has a tendency to

Table 8.2. FIGO staging of endometrial carcinoma

Stage I	
Ia G1,2,3	Tumour limited to the endometrium
Ib G1,2,3	Invasion of less than half of the myometrium
Ic G1,2,3	Invasion of more than half of the myometrium
Stage II	
IIa G1,2,3	Endocervical glandular involvement only
IIb G1,2,3	Cervical stromal invasion
Stage III	
IIIa G1,2,3	Tumour invades serosa and/or adenexae and/or malignant peritoneal cytology
IIIb G1,2,3	Vaginal metastases
IIIc G1,2,3	Metastases to pelvic and/or para-aortic lymph nodes
Stage IV	
IVa G1,2,3	Tumour invasion of the bladder and/or bowel mucosa
IVb	Distant metastases including intra-abdominal and/or inguinal lymph nodes

(continued)

Figure 8.2. (continued)
- A tissue sample or biopsy can be taken through some hysteroscopes. Alternatively, an endometrial biopsy device can be used, or the lining of the uterus can be scraped using an instrument called a curette (this is commonly known as a D&C). The tissue sample is sent for analysis.
- You may feel some discomfort similar to period pain for a few hours after hysteroscopy. You may also have a small amount of bleeding that lasts for 1–2 days.

Table 8.2. (continued)

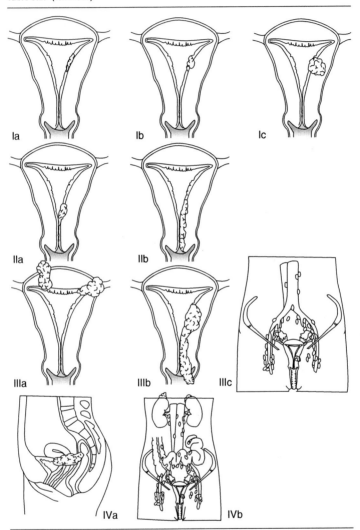

Ia   Ib   Ic

IIa   IIb

IIIa   IIIb   IIIc

IVa   IVb

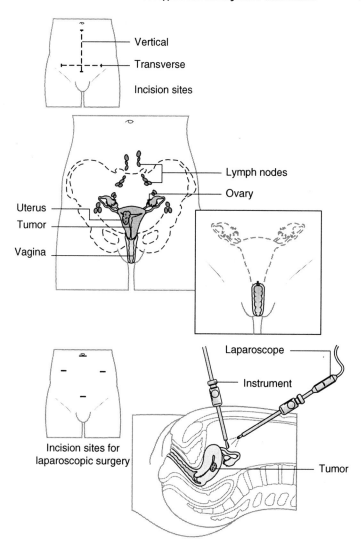

Figure 8.3. Hysterectomy for endometrial cancer

- The usual operation for endometrial cancer involves removing the uterus, cervix, both Fallopian tubes, and ovaries. The procedure is called a total abdominal hysterectomy and bilateral salpingo-oopherectomy (TAH & BSO).
- Sometimes it is also necessary to remove the fat "apron" in the abdomen (called the omentum), in a procedure called omentectomy. Similarly, the lymph glands in the pelvis may be removed.

pick up cancer cells, and if cancer develops in the omentum this means that there is spread outside the uterus and therefore the hysterectomy alone will not work as treatment.

For those women who have negative nodes, in other words, no spread to the lymph glands and no spread to the outside of the uterus, and where the muscle of the uterus (myometrium) is only invaded to less than 50% (Stages Ia and Ib), usually no further therapy is planned. For all more advanced stages, follow-up treatment with radiotherapy is standard.

Radiotherapy

When radiotherapy is given, it may be given intravaginally or through the abdomen. If you might be going for radiotherapy or wish to find out more about this, you may refer to Chapter 12.

Fertility Sparing Treatments for Endometrial Cancer

Until a few years ago, all of the treatments for endometrial cancer unfortunately involved loss of ability to have children, because the treatment always encompassed removing the uterus. However, in the last few years, for a woman who has no children and who presents to her gynecologist with an early-stage endometrial cancer, discussion may take place about other options. Any woman whose cancer is invading into the muscle of the uterus (Stage Ib or more) unfortunately and sadly still has no other option but to go forward with hysterectomy. However, for those women who have a Stage Ia cancer, in other words where the cancer is in the lining of the uterus, in the endometrium alone, it is possible to curette, or scrape the tumor off, and then commence progesterone therapy either in tablet form or, less likely, by the insertion of a Mirena™ device. It is very important to say that if your gynecologist starts this discussion with you, they will explain to you that the standard treatment has to remain hysterectomy for the time being. If, however, you have had no children,

---

Figure 8.3. (continued)

- The operation is carried out under general anesthetic, usually through a vertical (midline) or transverse (bikini-line) incision. A catheter may be passed up the urethra into the bladder to drain off the urine, and another tube may be inserted into the abdomen or vagina to drain any bleeding in the pelvis. These tubes may be left in place for 1–2 days.
- Sometimes, the hysterectomy is performed using keyhole surgery. A narrow telescope called a laparoscope is inserted though a small cut in the belly button. Keyhole surgery instruments are inserted into the abdomen through other small cuts in the abdominal wall. The laparoscope is used to perform the early steps of the hysterectomy, and the organs are finally removed through the vagina. Lymph glands in the pelvis can also be removed using the laparoscope.

you may wish to consider the progesterone therapy but it will be explained to you that there is a risk of cancer recurrence. As long as this happens within the uterus you will still have a curable disease. However, there are some women who develop secondary spread from endometrial cancer away from the uterus, for instance in the lungs. When the disease is in the lungs, cure is much less likely, and if you have gone down the route of sparing your fertility to discover that you have gone from having a curable cancer to a potentially incurable one, you would quite rightly feel devastated. These are very difficult choices for women to make and there is no doubting that the care you receive must be highly individualized. The risks, benefits, etc. must all be discussed with you in a clear fashion so that you know what to expect and what not to. For those women who undergo conservative therapy using progesterone drugs, re-hysteroscopy and resampling will take place on a very regular basis to make sure that if the cancer comes back it is hopefully detected early while it is still in the uterus and preferably at Stage I, and therefore curable by surgery alone.

For those women who are left without a uterus there has been much publicity around uterine transplantation and a number of groups of researchers (Giuseppe Del Priore and I are two) are involved in research in this area. It is, however, important to say that to date there are no successful uterine transplantations which have taken place in women. In a laboratory setting there have been some successes at performing the transplants, but a lack of success in terms of achieving pregnancies, and while I personally have little doubt that this type of operation will probably become available in the future, it is still many years off and it is in no way realistic to consider that this is on the immediate horizon.

Surgical procedures referred to in this chapter

Investigations	Hysteroscopy, dilatation and curettage
	Pipelle biopsy and ultrasound
Surgical treatment	Total abdominal hysterectomy and bilateral
	salpingo-oopherectomy (TAH, BSO)
	Laparoscopic TAH, BSO
	TAH, BSO, and lymph node sampling
	Radical lymphadenectomy and TAH, BSO
	Omentectomy

9. Vulval Cancer

General Facts

Vulval cancer is a rare cancer and accounts for only 3–5% of all malignancies in the sexual organs of women. It does appear to be getting commoner and does usually affect women who are elderly. Over half of the patients are above the age of 70. Having said this, about 15% of patients will be under the age of 40. The cause of vulval cancer is not fully understood, but it is known that some vulval cancers are preceded by a condition called vulval intraepithelial neoplasia (VIN). VIN is graded into 1, 2, and 3, and thus there is a sliding scale as shown in Figure 9.1. We also know that many women with VIN 1 spontaneously revert to normal. This can also happen with VIN 2 and 3, but usually these require treatment before it gets back to normal. We also know that VIN 2 and 3, if left untreated, would appear to have a high (perhaps 90%) chance of developing into vulval cancer, but over an extremely long period of time, probably on average 20–40 years. Unlike a similar condition in the cervix (cervical intraepithelial neoplasia [CIN]), which causes no symptoms, VIN tends to cause itching and discomfort; however, the vast majority of women who have itching and discomfort in the vulva have thrush and do not have VIN. Thrush is very common, VIN is very rare.

Other types of skin cancer can sometimes affect the vulva. These are usually dealt with by local removal (see Figure 9.1). VIN is treated either by excising the area as in Figure 9.1, or sometimes with laser treatment. As with all cancers, a staging system, i.e., a system that determines how far the cancer has spread, is used. Table 9.1 shows the various stages of vulval cancer, with pictures to illustrate each stage. Staging refers to how far the cancer has spread. It allows treatment to be tailored to you, the individual patient, and it allows different hospitals to compare results of different treatments. **The FIGO staging I–IV has no relationship with four cusps A–D.**

Diagnosis

You might probably have noticed a lump on the outside of your vagina, or have itching or discomfort, or occasionally bleeding or bad smelling discharge, which would have made you go to your doctor. Your doctor might have

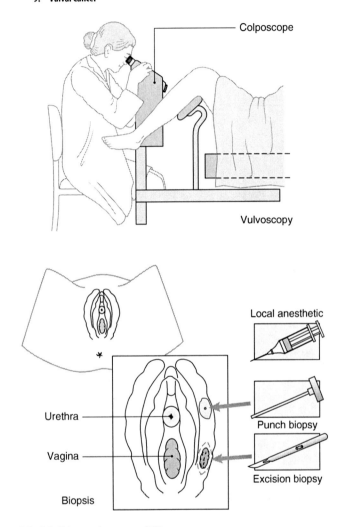

Figure 9.1. Vulval biopsy and treatment of VIN

- To diagnose vulval intraepithelial neoplasia (VIN), the vulva is examined in a procedure called vulvoscopy. A special microscope called a colposcope is usually used. Vulvoscopy is a painless, outpatient procedure. You will be asked to lie on your back with your legs in supports.

- Dilute acetic acid may be painted onto your vulva to show up any abnormal cells. This is not painful, but may cause mild irritation.

- Samples of vulval tissue, called vulval biopsies, may be removed for examination in the laboratory. These are taken either after numbing the area with local anesthetic or under a general anesthetic. Your doctor may take several small circular punch biopsies (tiny circular samples of skin), or remove a larger piece of tissue (called an excision biopsy). You will probably need a few stitches after an excision biopsy, and these will leave a small scar.

examined you and referred you to a gynecologist. You might have been referred to a colposcopy clinic (colposcopy is microscopic examination of the cervix and vagina and this can also include microscopic examination of the outside of the vagina, i.e., the vulva). The golden rule with all lumps or ulcers on the vulva is that if there is no infection diagnosed, then your doctor must take a sample to exclude a diagnosis of VIN or vulval cancer. Warts on the vulva are very common, but it is important that, if you have warts, once they have been treated you are examined to make sure they have gone. The sample from the vulva may be taken either in the outpatient clinic using local anesthetic, or it may be done in the operating theater with you under a general anesthetic, depending upon the size of sample that one wishes to obtain. Figure 9.1 shows the device used in the outpatient clinic, which removes a very small sample of tissue. If you have had a diagnosis of VIN as stated above, the treatment will be some form of local therapy to remove the area, either by lasering it or excising it.

Table 9.1. Tumor-node-metastasis (TNM) staging of vulval carcinoma

Stage 0	Carcinoma in situ, intraepithelial carcinoma
Stage I	Lesions of 2 cm or less confined to the vulva or perineum. Absence of lymph node metastases
Ia	Lesions of 2 cm or less in size, confined to the vulva or perineum with stromal invasion to a depth of no more than 1 mm. No nodal metastases
Ib	Lesions of 2 cm or less in size, confined to the vulva or perineum with stromal invasion to a depth greater than 1 mm. No nodal metastasis
Stage II	Tumor confined to the vulva and/or perineum, or more than 2 cm at its greatest dimension. No nodal metastases
Stage III	Tumor of any size on the vulva and/or perineum with:
	1. Adjacent spread to the lower urethra and/or the vagina or the anus and/or
	2. Unilateral regional lymph node metastases
Stage IV	
IVa	Tumor invading any of the following: upper urethra, bladder mucosa, rectal mucosa, pelvic bone, and/or bilateral regional node metastases
IVb	Any distant metastases including pelvic lymph nodes

Used with the permission of the American Joint Committee on Cancer (AJCC), Chicago, Illinois. The original source for this material is the AJCC Cancer Staging Manual, Sixth Edition (2002) published by Springer Science and Business Media LLC, www.springerlink.com

Figure 9.1. (continued)
    If you have VIN, the abnormal cells may be removed, or sometimes destroyed using a laser. This is usually carried out under general anesthetic. You will be given painkillers and possibly also a local anesthetic jelly to use for a few days after treatment.
- After VIN has been diagnosed, you will require regular vulvoscopy. An alternative way of managing this condition is to remove only areas that appear to be progressing towards early cancer. This may save unnecessary surgery.

Table 9.1. (continued)

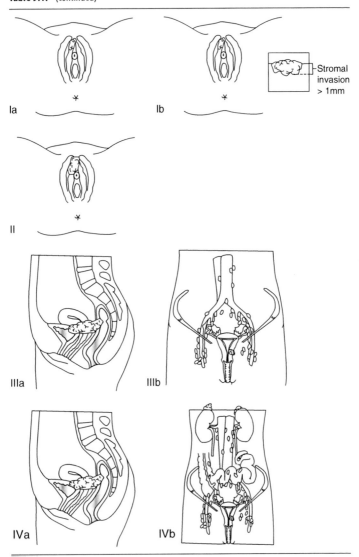

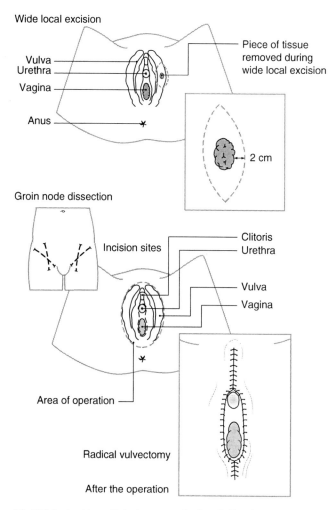

Wide local excision

Vulva
Urethra
Vagina

Anus

Piece of tissue
removed during
wide local excision

2 cm

Groin node dissection

Incision sites

Clitoris
Urethra

Vulva
Vagina

Area of operation

Radical vulvectomy

After the operation

Figure 9.2. Wide local excision, radical vulvectomy, and groin node dissection

- If you have a small vulval cancer, it may be removed under general anesthetic in a procedure called wide local excision. A small amount of normal surrounding tissue is also removed. Unless the cancer is at a very early stage, the lymph glands in one or both groins are also removed.
- You may be monitored with vulvoscopy up to four times a year to check that the cancer has not returned.
- If the cancer is more advanced, an operation called radical vulvectomy and groin node dissection is usually required. This involves removing the entire vulva and the lymph glands in the groins. If necessary, the lower part of the urethra can be removed without affecting bladder function. The skin with the pubic hair is not normally removed.

Vulval Cancer

If the diagnosis is that there is a cancer present, you will have a number of tests performed. These will include checking your blood count to make sure that you are not anemic, checking your blood salts (urea and electrolytes) and liver function tests, you will have a chest x-ray, and since you are likely to require an anesthetic you will have an electrocardiograph (ECG). Usually some forms of scanning will be performed and because these cancers can sometimes spread to the lymph nodes, ultrasound may well be performed of the lymph nodes. Sometimes samples are taken from the lymph nodes using a fine needle. This is also done under local anesthetic. Sometimes a magnetic resonance imaging (MRI) or computed tomography (CT) scan is also done.

The treatment for vulval cancers used to be in the form of very disfiguring surgery, but mercifully that has all now changed. The drawing shown in Figure 9.2 shows the incisions used if the lymph nodes need to be removed and, as you can see, these leave two almost invisible scars in the groin. Some centers now offer a new technique called sentinel node biopsy to reduce the number of lymph nodes requring removal. With respect to the vulva itself, it partly depends on how big the area is that needs to be removed and its exact position. If it is on one side or the other it is usually possible just to excise the area of the tumor along with an area of normal tissue around it. If the clitoris is not involved with the tumor, great efforts are made to preserve as much normal tissue as possible, so that sexual function will be as normal as possible afterwards. Cosmetically, it is obvious that the less the tissue is removed, the better is the result. Having said this, even when a lot of tissue has to be removed, people are usually very surprised at the acceptability of the result once everything has healed up.

For those people who have Stage 1 and Stage 2, the cure rates are very high. You will be followed up after your operation and seen every 3–4 months for the first couple of years and then probably every 6 months for the next 3 years, and then probably once a year thereafter until 10 years after treatment. Radiotherapy is sometimes required if the lymph nodes are involved and further details with respect to radiotherapy can be found in Chapter 12.

Figure 9.2.   (continued)
- The operation is carried out under general anesthetic, usually though separate cuts in the groins and around the vulva. The skin at the bottom of the vagina is stitched directly to the skin outside the vulva. Tubes drain lymph fluid from the groin wounds for up to 10 days after surgery.
- Depending on the pathology report, you may require radiotherapy after the wounds have healed. You will be seen regularly at the clinic for at least 5–10 years. Penetrative sex is usually, but not always, possible after a radical vulvectomy. If not, reconstructive surgery may be possible at a later date.

Sexual Function

It is thought that there are four types of women, in terms of orgasmic function: Those who achieve deep vaginal orgasms, those who achieve orgasm by superficial clitoral stimulation and external genital stimulation, those who have both, and those who have neither. Operations on the vulva do not have any effect on the vaginal type of orgasm, but if the clitoris is removed and/or the labia minoria, it may have an effect on your ability to achieve an external stimulation orgasm. This is part of the reason, as well as the cosmetics of it, for trying to preserve as much tissue as possible. You should discuss this sort of thing with your gynecologist if you are sexually active, or you may feel more comfortable discussing this with the specialist nurse if you prefer.

10. Breast Cancer

Introduction

Breast cancer is the commonest form of cancer in women in western countries and accounts for 18% of all cancers in women. In the UK there are approximately 25,000 new cases diagnosed every year and sadly there are around 15,000 deaths every year. Breast cancer is still the leading cause of death among women aged between 35 and 55 years. 50% occurs in the 50–60 age group and 30% in those over the age of 70.

On the positive side, results of breast cancer treatment continue to improve and with new targeted drug treatments along with the use of molecular markers it is likely that there will be much more accuracy in treatment with tailoring of the treatment to meet your individual needs. In the last 10 years in the UK breast cancer deaths have fallen by 22%. This probably reflects improved screening coupled with improved treatments and delivery of those treatments. One very recent study also showed the benefits of chemotherapy on reducing the rate of cancers returning over a 28-year follow-up with no deleterious effects from that chemotherapy. Similarly, we know that those women who are prescribed tamoxifen definitely benefit from it in the long term, making its side effects worth putting up with.

Breast cancer varies depending upon where one lives. It is common in North America and Western Europe, and uncommon in Asia and Africa. Genetic factors also appear to be important. In terms of judging risk, the risk is greatest by far in those over the age of 50 and very unlikely in those under the age of 30. It is much commoner in women who have two first-degree relatives, i.e., their mother or sister with breast cancer diagnosed at an early age, or in a woman who has had cancer in one breast it is much more likely to occur in the other. Much has been written in the newspapers about the genetic effect although overall about 10–15% of breast cancers are in fact attributable to family history. The longer one has periods, the higher is the risk; in other words, an early start to periods and a late menopause increases the risks as does being over weight. Taking the oral contraceptive pill appears to greatly reduce the risk of ovarian and endometrial cancers, but causes a slightly increased risk in breast cancer, but this risk goes away once you are 10 years beyond stopping the pill. An enormous amount has been written on the risks associated with hormone replacement therapy (Table 10.1).

Table 10.1. Summary of the risks and benefits associated with using HRT.

Condition	Age of woman (yr)	Number of cases per 1000 non-HRT users	Extra number of cases in 1000 HRT users over the same period	
			5 years use	**10 years use**
Cumlative cancer risk over 15 Or 20 years				
Breast cancer	50–65	32	1.5 (±1.5) oestrogen-only 6 (±1) (combined HRT)	5 (±2) oestrogen-only 19 (±1) (combined HRT)
Endometrial cancer	50–64	5	4 (oestrogen-only) Data not available for combined HRT	10 (oestrogen-only) 2* (combined HRT)
Ovarian cancer[b]	50–69	9	1 (±1) (oestrogen-only)	3 (±2) (oestrogen-only)
Cardiovascular risks over 5 years				
Stroke	50–59	3	1 (±1)	Data not available
	60–69	11	4 (±3)	
VTE	50–59	3	4 (±2)	Data not available
	60–69	8	9 (±5)	
Benifits over 5 years			**Reduced number of cases in 1000 HRT users over the same period**	
Colorectal cancer	50–59	3	1 (±1)	2 (±2)
	60–69	8	3 (±2)	5-6 (±4)
Fracture of neck of femue	50–59	1–2	0–1 (±1)	1 (±1)
	60–69	7–8	2–3 (±2)	5 (±3)

Numbers are best estimates (± approximate range from 95% Confidence Intervals).

*There may be a difference in the risk of endometrial cancer between sequential and continuous combined HRT.

In summary, age is the greatest risk factor while carrying the breast cancer gene BRCA1 and BRCA2 denotes higher risk, but actually accounts for only a small proportion of woman getting cancer. Although given maximum media coverage hormone replacement therapy (HRT) certainly in the first 5 years of usage probably confers minimal risk.

Screening

Currently in the UK breast cancer screening starts at age 50 and is undertaken on a three-yearly basis by mammography. Mammograms are done by taking x-rays of breast tissue. The breast is compressed between two plates, which can sometimes cause discomfort particularly if you have small breasts. In North America and other Western European countries mammogram screening often starts at age 40 and in women with a strong family history, particularly where relatives have been affected at a young age, it may start at age 35.

This partly stems from women's perception of risk of breast cancer. It is true that as a bald statistic 1 in 12 women will develop breast cancer; however, this is a risk which takes into account women right through to age 85 and in real terms the risk for women aged between 30 and 50 is 1:1,000 per year, while under the age of 30 is almost negligible. The risk between age 50 and 70 when mammography is advised in the UK is 2:1,000 per year. These statistics contrast strongly with patient surveys which show that women overestimate the risk of dying from breast cancer in the next 10 years by 22 times and overestimate the benefit of screening by 127 times. It is therefore fair to say that in strict cost benefits terms the UK screening program is ideal, although in terms of helping women come to terms with their risk there may be advantages in starting screening at age 40, perhaps with 1–2-yearly screening from 40 to 50 and two-yearly from 50 onwards.

Figure 10.1 is a drawing of the breast showing the various structures within it. Figure 10.2 alongside shows where breast cancers themselves arise and these very rarely arise in the breast tissue, which is not the glandular tissue; in other

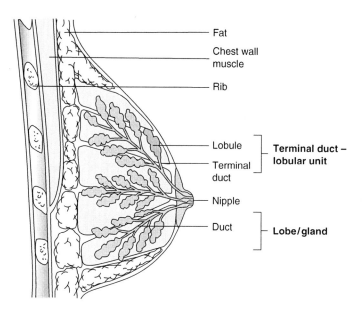

Figure 10.1. "Breast anatomy" (Courtesy Health Press. Baum H, Schipper H, Breast Cancer, 2nd Edition)

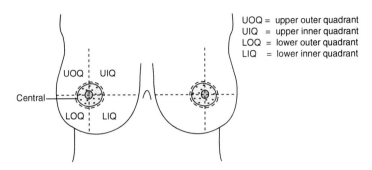

UOQ = upper outer quadrant
UIQ = upper inner quadrant
LOQ = lower outer quadrant
LIQ = lower inner quadrant

Figure 10.2. Possible sites of tumor

words, the tissue that is designed to make milk. Of all the breast lumps discovered 80% are benign but naturally cause a lot of anxiety. The benign causes include fibroadenomas, simple cysts, infection, and problems that women are born with. In addition, bruising can cause a collection of blood which can feel like a lump.

However, for a woman who has a breast cancer this will be staged. The most widely used classification of breast cancer is the tumor-nodes-metastases (TNM) classification. **This staging, T (tumor) 0–4, N (node) 0–3, and M (metastasis) 0–1, does not in any way relate to the four cusps (A–D).**

There is also the Union Internationale Contre Cancer (UICC) staging system for breast cancer, which incorporates the TNM classification. Again this has no relationship to the four cusps (A–D).

UICC stage TNM classification

I	T1, N0, M0
II	T1, N1, M0; T2, N0–1, M0*
III	Any, T, N2–3, M0; T3, any N, M0; T4 any N, M0
IV	Any T, any N, M1

Many expert groups include T2 tumors in Stage 1.

Breast Self-examination

Breast self-examination has long been promoted as a way to promote earlier detection of cancers, but as can been seen if 80% of lumps are benign, then much anxiety is caused by breast examination being done by you. Instead of breast examination breast awareness is now being promoted, which is encouraging woman to be aware of their breasts and if they develop dimpling or flaking of the skin, unusual pain or discomfort, nipple discharge, lumps, or thickening, which is not cyclical and any new appearance to their breasts, then they should go to see their doctor. This may well be more helpful than performing systematic examination of your breasts on a regular basis.

Once You or Your Doctor Find a Lump

Once this has happened you will be referred to a specialist who will do what is called a triple assessment, which will involve examining you and asking you many questions, then using some form of x-ray, ultrasound, or magnetic resonance imaging (MRI) techniques to further visualize the lump and also to look at the lymph glands in the armpits. In Europe fine-needle aspiration cytology is often done (see Figure 10.3). This is less common in North America where biopsies are more currently undertaken (Figure 10.4). These techniques allow the diagnosis to be made and the stage of the tumor as previously shown in Table 10.2 to be worked out. The treatment which you will be offered depends on whether the cancer is thought to be curable and therefore usually an early cancer or a late cancer which is much less likely to be cured. Therefore I have divided the next bit into two sections reflecting these two groups and the different goals of treatment.

Management of Early Cancer

The goal of the treatment is to prevent or delay recurrence of the cancer for as long as possible. The idea is to accomplish this with the minimum of surgery, minimum of chemotherapy, minimum of hormone therapy, and minimum of radiotherapy; in other words, to give the best cure rate with the least side affects. Currently, most women will start their treatment with surgery and

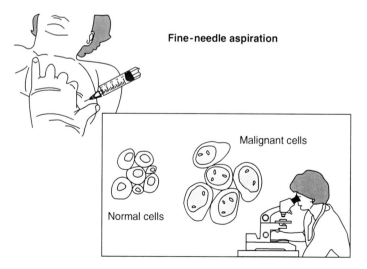

Figure 10.3. Fine-needle aspiration

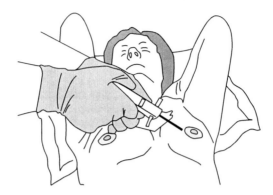

Figure 10.4. Core biopsy of a breast lump

Table 10.2. Tumor status

T0	No palpable tumor
T1	Tumor 2 cm with no fixation*
T2	Tumor >2 cm but <5 cm with no fixation*
T3	Tumor maximum diameter >5 cm with no fixation[a]
T4	Tumor of any size with either fixation to chest wall or ulceration of skin
Status of lymph nodes	
N0	No palpable axillary nodes
N1a	Palpable nodes not thought to contain tumor
N1b	Palpable nodes thought to contain tumor
N2	Nodes >2 cm or fixed to one another and deep structures
N3	Supraclavicular or infraclavicular nodes
Distant metastases	
M0	No clinically apparent distant metastases
M1	Distant metastases obvious

[a]*For T1–T3 "a" indicates no attachment to underlying muscles; "b" indicates attachment*
Used with the permission of the American Joint Committee on Cancer (AJCC), Chicago, Illinois.
The original source for this material is the AJCC Cancer Staging Manual, Sixth Edition (2002)
published by Springer Science and Business Media LLC, www.springerlink.com

then move onto some form of either hormone therapy or chemotherapy. However, there is little evidence to support surgery being the first line of treatment and on occasion this order may be reversed. In terms of the surgical options for breast cancer these are conservative surgery, in other words where the lump itself is just removed. This has the advantage of retaining the breast and the disadvantage of making it slightly more difficult to monitor in the longer term. The other option is removal of the breast (simple mastectomy). This usually means that radiotherapy is not required to the breast but may still be required to the armpit and then there are forms of radical mastectomy which are now much less common. Figures 10.5–10.8 demonstrate these procedures.

After removal of the breast you could develop some complications, which include bruising, swelling, delayed healing, infection, and a damaged brachial nerve; this can cause numbness in the arm. Fortunately this is uncommon. In addition to this, shoulder weakness and/or stiffness and swelling of the arm can occasionally occur.

In general, for breast cancer to be suitable for conservative surgery there should only be one lump and it should be less than or equal to 4 cm in diameter with no metastases. In other words, there must be no known spread of the cancer out of your breast.

The other vexed issue is what to do about the lymph nodes since removing these often increases the side effects associated with the surgery. Until recently, the lymph nodes were usually removed and mostly they were found not to have cancer in them, so that in retrospect it seemed to have been the wrong thing to do to have removed them. This is particularly the case since removal of lymph nodes can lead to swelling in the arm and discomfort (lymphedema). The management of lymphedema is described elsewhere (pages 101–103).

In contrast, it was considered too dangerous to take a chance and not to remove the lymph nodes, since if they did had cancer in them and were not removed the cure rate fell sharply.

Much research has gone into trying to identify whether nodes were involved prior to surgery to reduce the number of unnecessary lymph node removals.

Breast Lumpectomy/wide local excision

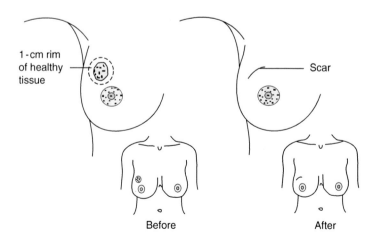

Figure 10.5. Breast Lumpectomy/wide local excision

Quadrantectomy

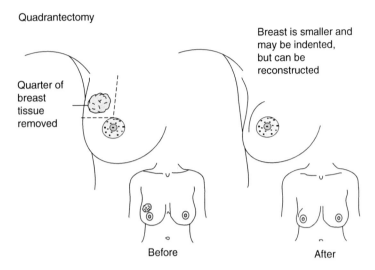

Quarter of
breast
tissue
removed

Breast is smaller and
may be indented,
but can be
reconstructed

Before   After

Figure 10.6. Removal of part of the breast.

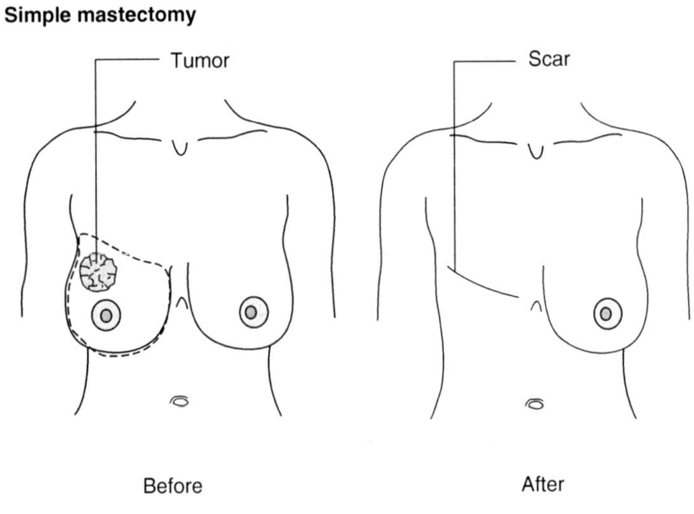

Simple mastectomy

Tumor   Scar

Before   After

Figure 10.7. Simple mastectomy/removal of the whole breast

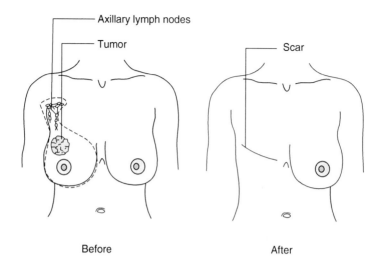

Figure 10.8. Modified radical mastectomy: removal of breast and axillary (armpit) tissue

One of the difficulties is that x-ray techniques such as computed tomography (CT) scanning, MRI, or ultrasound can only detect lymph node involvement once the nodes are heavily involved with tumor. If there is only microscopic, in other words not visible to the naked eye, involvement of the nodes with cancer, then the x-ray techniques are poor.

Recently, the new technology of sentinel lymph node biopsy has become available. This allows for removal of just one node to check whether there has been any spread. If there has not, then it is reasonable to assume that the other nodes are not involved with cancer. If the sentinel node is positive, then you can assume that the other nodes are at high risk of involvement and therefore their removal is necessary. This has helped to greatly reduce the number of complete lymph node removals (lymphadenectomies) being undertaken. I think one of the very difficult things for women to cope with in the past was that they had got bad side effects from the lymph node removal and that it had not been necessary anyway. Now at least if it has to be done and you do get side effects, at least you know that was strictly necessary to improve the chances of cure.

Nowadays reconstructive surgery is also possible and there are many different ways of doing this. It may be done at the same time as your initial operation or it may be done later. These are all issues you should discuss with your surgeon or your breast cancer specialist.

Radiotherapy

Most women will have radiotherapy after their surgery if they have had conservative surgery, in other words the lump only removed, and the treatment that is given is usually 3–5 times per week for 6 weeks. Radiotherapy can give side affects in the form of nausea, vomiting, skin rashes, and occasional inflammation of the lung. It has however been shown to reduce the chances of local recurrence of the disease in breast-conserving surgery by 20–30% over a 10-year period.

In terms of other treatments, chemotherapy has commonly been used in women under the age of 50 and tamoxifen or aromatase therapy in women over the age of 50. It would however appear that perhaps much of the benefit of chemotherapy in women under the age of 50 is in the effect that the chemotherapy has on the ovaries by making the ovaries become menopausal, i.e., stopping them working, and that this effect can also be got from the use of other drugs designed to stop the ovaries functioning. These are given by injection, either monthly or three-monthly (e.g., GnRH analogue). Particularly, drugs can have an advantage if you are a younger woman looking to have children in the future. A woman over the age of 50 appears to be best benefited from tamoxifen, but it does have side effects of giving menopause symptoms, in other words flushes and sweats and very occasionally endometrial cancer. This has been much hyped up by the press and the risk of endometrial cancer is 1:1,000 with 5 years worth of treatment. However, tamoxifen reduces the risk of death from breast cancer by 20–30%. In other words, if your doctor has suggested you take tamoxifen, you should take it as the advantage would appear to be very high. Sometimes there is no point taking tamoxifen if your tumor has not got any oestrogen receptor, or if it has not got the right factors in the breast to make the tamoxifen work. Your breast tissue which was removed would be analyzed for both estrogen and progesterone receptors, the two common female hormones to help tailor the treatment appropriately. Newer drugs known as aromatase inhibitors also look as if they are producing promising results. In terms of the problems of chemotherapy please refer to Chapter 12.

Much has been written with respect to hormone replacement therapy for survivors of breast cancer and this can be a very vexed issue. However, it is certainly fair to say that breast cancer is not an absolute counterindication to taking hormone replacement therapy and it should be judged upon the symptoms, depending upon the symptoms that you yourself are suffering from.

Management of Advanced Cancer

The goal of the treatment here is unfortunately not to achieve cure, but to give you the best quality of life possible with the minimum side effects from the treatment which is suggested. The treatment may incorporate chemotherapy, hormone (endocrine) therapy, surgery, and radiotherapy, depending upon where your disease is. If the disease is in the bone, there are good responses from radiotherapy, which can give very good relief of symptoms, the principle symptom of course being pain. Readers are referred to Chapter 13 on management of pain. The one thing that is not covered in this chapter which is specific for breast cancer, bone pain, is the use of a new class of drugs called bisphosphonates, which are very good for controlling the calcium levels in the blood stream and can be very good for pain associated with secondary cancer in the bone.

Sex and Body Image

While the new approaches with smaller operations, less removal of lymph nodes, and better reconstructive surgery have all greatly helped, women are still to greater or lesser degrees traumatized by their diagnosis, treatment, and the uncertainties which the future holds. In general terms, Chapter 15 on grief is worth reading because it goes through the range of emotions you will experience in the wake of your diagnosis. Specific issues with respect to sex and body image can often be addressed by counseling, psychotherapeutic interventions, and complementary techniques such as self-hypnosis. These are described in Chapter 14.

How Do I Cope with My Diagnosis and Disease

If you have breast cancer which has been detected early and treated where the goal has been to achieve cure, you will be followed up on a regular basis with examinations to check the breast and intermittent blood tests and x-rays. The evidence to support this sort of follow-up is not particularly strong, although it is designed to decrease anxiety, not to increase it. One of the great difficulties with all cancers is the fear that it will come back, and breast cancer like all other cancers can come back and unfortunately, slightly differently from many of the pelvic cancers, it can come back after many years. In other words, all is well for many years and then it can reappear. Most of the other cancers described in

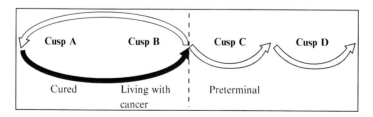

Figure 10.9.

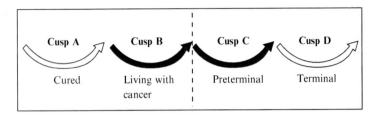

Figure 10.10.

this book, if they have gone for 5 years, are very unlikely to reappear. Psychologically, therefore, if you are in the group where cure has been aimed at it is a bit like a mixture of cusps A and B (Figure 10.9). If you are in the group where cure is not achievable, then cusps B and C are where you are (see Figure 10.10). Readers are referred to Chapter 3. Chapter 16 on spirituality again may make for useful reference.

Useful Addresses

www.adjuvantsite.com
(program for estimation of risk and benefits of adjuvant therapy)

www.minervation.com/cancer/breast/professional/
(UK National Electronic Library for Health information on breast cancer)

CancerBACUP
3,Bath Place
Rivington Street
London, EC2A 3JR
Tel: 0808 800 1234
http://www.cancerbacup.org.uk/

Cancer Research UK
PO Box 123
Lincoln's Inn Fields
London, WC2A 3PX
Tel: 020 7242 0200
Fax: 02 07269 3100
www.cancerresearchuk.org/aboutcancer/specificcancers/93645
http://www.crc.org.uk/cancer/Aboutcan_common2.html

11. Choriocarcinoma: Gestational Trophoblastic Neoplasia

General Facts

This condition describes a whole spectrum of diseases which include hydatidiform mole, invasive mole, choriocarcinoma, and placental site tumor. Up until about 40 years ago, if a diagnosis of choriocarcinoma was made for a patient, the cure rate was sadly very low. Fortunately, this has now radically changed and choriocarcinoma is one of the most curable of gynecological cancers. Hydatidiform moles are not cancers and invasive moles act somewhat like cancers. As with many other cancers, there is a sliding scale in terms of "aggressiveness," hydatidiform mole is a local problem, whereas a choriocarcinoma or placental site tumor can be a disseminated problem; in other words, it can spread through the body. Your chances of being cured with this condition are very high, even if it has spread, either by using surgery or chemotherapy, or sometimes radiotherapy. Many women, after treatment for this condition, go on to have children.

Hydatidiform Mole

The incidence of this condition varies depending upon where one lives. In the UK and the USA it occurs in about 1 in 1,200 pregnancies, but in the Far East it affects 1 in 77 pregnancies in some areas. It is also related to the age of the mother. The lowest chance of occurrence is when you become pregnant between 20 and 29 years of age and the highest chance is if you become pregnant when you are under the age of 15 or over the age of 40. The condition does not appear to be related to whether you have had children before, what kind of contraception you have used, or if you have had radiotherapy or chemotherapy in the past.

Hydatidiform moles are classified as either complete or partial. The complete type carries a higher chance of progressing to an invasive mole or choriocarcinoma than the partial type. If you have a complete mole, you have approximately a 7% chance that you will need chemotherapy, whereas if you have a partial mole, the chance is 3%. The partial mole accounts for approximately 15% of all cases.

All of these conditions are part of an abnormality associated with pregnancy and they produce a positive pregnancy test. Pregnancy tests measure the levels of the hormone beta human chorionic gonadotrophin (beta hCG), which is normally produced by the placenta during normal pregnancy. Most pregnancy tests bought in pharmacies give either a positive or a negative result. In hospital, however, pregnancy tests performed on blood give either a negative result or, if positive, give a sliding scale from weakly positive to highly positive. Usually very early in pregnancy the test is weakly positive and over the first 12 weeks it gets more positive, before subsiding thereafter. In choriocarcinoma, the blood test is very strongly positive. Ironically, although the beta HCG levels may be very high the urine pregnancy test may be negative. The reason that the blood test is strongly positive is because the hormone beta HCG is raised. This is the hormone which causes feelings of nausea and morning sickness in early pregnancy. If you have a hydatidiform mole you may have exaggerated symptoms, i.e., lots of early morning sickness etc., in the early part of the pregnancy. In a normal pregnancy half of the genetic content of the baby comes from the man and half from the woman. The man's half is contained within the sperm and the woman's half within the egg produced in the ovary. Where a complete mole has developed an empty egg is fertilized by the male sperm and the complete genetic content is male only. There is no baby, no fetus and only an afterbirth which is a grape-like substance that fills the uterus. In the partial mole, a fetus is present. Instead of there being the normal two sets of chromosomes, there are three sets of chromosomes and the fetus dies usually in the first few weeks of pregnancy.

Usually you will have noticed that your periods have stopped and you felt pregnant, or perhaps there might have been bleeding suggesting a miscarriage. Very occasionally, people see the grape-like things passing from their vagina along with the blood. Sometimes the condition can also cause the blood pressure to be raised and the thyroid gland in the neck to be overactive. Nowadays, the diagnosis is usually made at ultrasound scanning, but sometimes the diagnosis is made following evacuation of the uterus because of either a suspected miscarriage or termination of pregnancy. Because the molar tissue secretes beta hCG, even after you have had an evacuation, the pregnancy test will remain positive and the signs of pregnancy which you may have felt, may well continue. Treatment for hydatidiform mole is by removing the contents from the uterus (Figure 11.1). This may have to be done on two occasions to completely empty the uterus and your gynecologist may do this with the help of an ultrasound machine on your tummy to confirm that the uterus has been emptied.

If you have had a diagnosis of a hydatidiform mole made and then confirmed with evacuation of your uterus, the decision as to whether you need any more treatment is based upon the following:

- Your beta hCG level, which will be measured every 1–2 weeks until it is negative on two occasions. It will be measured every 2 months for a year and you will be advised to use contraception, other than the combined oral contraceptive pill, for 6–12 months. In addition, physical examination is carried out, including examination of the vagina, cervix, and uterus, every 3 months for a year. You will also have a chest x-ray done, which, assuming it is normal, is reassuring.

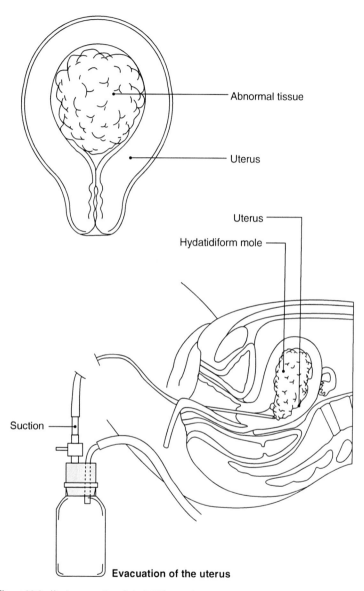

Figure 11.1. Uterine evacuation of a hydatidiform mole

- If, however, your beta HCG level stops going down or rises, or there was anything detected by way of spread of the molar tissue, then you would be started on chemotherapy immediately.

Gestational Trophoblastic Neoplasia

Gestational trophoblastic neoplasia (GTN) is classified into Stage 1, where there is no evidence of disease spread outside the uterus, and Stage 2, where there is disease spread outside the uterus. Stage 2 is divided into A and B. A is where there is what is referred to as "good prognosis metastatic disease" and B is where there is "poor prognosis metastatic disease."

The risk of recurrence of gestational trophoblastic neoplasia in those people who have no spread outside the uterus is negligible as the success of treatment is virtually 100%. Where there is "good prognosis spread outside the uterus," again there is close to 100% success of treatment and where the prognosis is regarded as poor and there is disease outside the uterus, the success rate still remains high, in the region of 70%. Another way of looking at this is that the chance of the disease recurring, if there is no spread outside the uterus, is 2.1%; if there is good prognosis spread outside the uterus it is 5.4% and if there is poor prognosis outside the uterus it is 21%. Where recurrence happens, re-treatment is feasible and for a very small minority of women, further surgery may be required. This combination of treatments makes it very unlikely that women with gestational trophoblastic neoplasia will be anything other than cured of their disease. In addition, the vast majority will retain their fertility.

General Treatments and Care

12. General Concepts of Chemotherapy and Radiotherapy

Chemotherapy can be used in most of the cancers that affect women's gynecological organs, although chemotherapy is most commonly used for women who have ovarian cancer. There are lots of misconceptions that people have about chemotherapy. First, and most important, is that I often hear people say that it probably does not work. This is simply just not true. The difficulty with chemotherapy is in some ways having a picture in one's mind's eye of what a cancer is like and then imagining a drug being poured in (usually in a drip and into a vein), so how can this possibly get rid of the cancer? As a surgeon I wholeheartedly and rightly believe in the type of treatment that I offer. It is also true that it is easier, I think, for the patient to visualize a cancer being cut out and therefore it is removed, whereas it is difficult to see how a drug can do anything other than perhaps just shrink things down. I can quite honestly personally testify to having looked inside lots of people's tummies before and after chemotherapy and the difference is truly staggering. Lots and lots of tumors just literally disappear into thin air after chemotherapy.

What is true about chemotherapy is that it varies in its effectiveness. Partly, this is down to whether the tumor is sensitive to the chemotherapy which is being prescribed, and if it is sensitive, how sensitive is it? Some people will have very little response to chemotherapy and some will have a huge response. The response of the majority will lie somewhere between these two extremes. The difficulty is that one never knows what response one will make until one has taken the chemotherapy.

In practical terms, chemotherapy usually involves going to the medical day unit or perhaps being admitted to the ward for 1 day every 1–3 weeks, depending upon what is being given. A drip is put up (see picture) and the drug is given through this drip over the course of the day. Various blood tests have to be taken as the chemotherapy progresses to make sure that there are no untoward side effects developing. People worry greatly about the side effects, particularly nausea and vomiting, and while these do still occur, they are not nearly as severe as they used to be, partly because the drugs have become more refined, but also because there are newer drugs which can be given to stop feelings of nausea and vomiting. Probably the biggest worry in terms of side effects is hair loss, which for most women is a very disturbing side effect. There are, however, many groups of drugs which do not involve hair loss and for those that do, it is very important to say that hair will grow back after the treatment has finished and often more luxuriantly than it was before. Strangely, some people who have curly hair grow it back straight and some people with straight hair grow back curly hair. This sort of feature is quite unpredictable. What is completely predictable is that the hair will grow back.

Another side effect is that of feeling tired, and there is no doubting that as the treatments progress people begin to feel much more tired. One of my own friends who had chemotherapy was able to come around to my house for dinner after the first "pulse" of chemotherapy. Each time you come in for a treatment, this is referred to as a "pulse" and as each pulse is given, people tend to feel progressively more tired. The friend I mentioned above was able to come around for dinner to eat a hearty meal, washed down with a couple of glasses of wine, without feeling in any way unwell.

An unusual side effect can be peripheral neuropathy, which can cause troublesome symptoms including tingling, burning, and pain in the limbs including hands and feet. These and the treatments available are discussed in Chapter 13.

Chemotherapy tends to be given in a number of pulses, usually five as a minimum or 12 as a maximum, although this will very much depend upon what drug is being given for what condition (see Figure 12.1). For those who

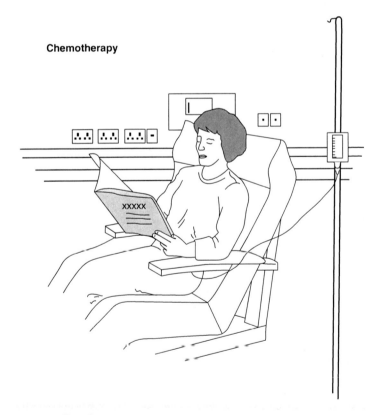

Figure 12.1. Chemotherapy

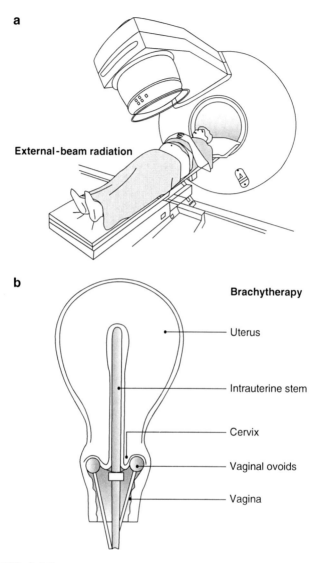

a

External-beam radiation

b

Brachytherapy

Uterus

Intrauterine stem

Cervix

Vaginal ovoids

Vagina

Figure 12.2. Radiotherapy

have cancer in the vagina or cervix, chemotherapy may be given as treatment alongside radiotherapy and this is to maximize the chances of cure. It fulfils the maxim we discussed earlier, namely that you should always hit cancers hard and fast, and hitting a cancer with both radiotherapy and chemotherapy can sometimes be more effective than one of these treatments alone.

Radiotherapy can either be used as the main treatment for gynecological cancers or can be used as an addition following surgery or chemotherapy. Again, with radiotherapy, it is often difficult to visualize exactly how a tumor can be cured and made to completely disappear, when you feel nothing and see nothing during the treatments, but very many tumors are cured.

Radiotherapy involves the use of equipment which delivers a dose of radiation to a specific site. The radiation may be given from an external source or it may be given internally, with a device placed inside the vagina (see Figure 12.2). Occasionally rods may be placed into the tumor to allow direct access of the radiotherapy into the middle of the cancer itself. How the radiotherapy is given depends upon where the cancer is, and you should look at the specific chapter, e.g., cervix or vagina, etc., to see the likely method for radiotherapy in your case. In general, radiotherapy is given as a course, where it is given Monday to Friday for a number of weeks. This involves coming to the hospital for a meeting when the whole treatment plan is decided. Thereafter, when you come to the hospital you are only there for a few minutes, having the treatment, and then you go home again. You do not actually feel anything at all as the treatment itself is taking place, but over the weeks you may well find that you feel very tired. In addition, you can sometimes get urinary upset with cystitis type symptoms and some bowel symptoms, which can alternate between diarrhea and constipation and sometimes colicky pain. Very occasionally you can get pain and tingling in the skin and sometimes a burning sensation in the skin. All of these things are treatable and some of the treatments are discussed in Chapter 13.

Radiotherapy like surgery causes long-term scarring, which can cause longer-term bowel and bladder upset. If you are troubled by symptoms you should tell your doctor since there are usually effective remedies available. It can also result in vaginal narrowing and dryness. Both of these can create difficulty in having sex including discomfort, pain, and bleeding. Graduated dilators and creams can give much relief of symptoms and occasionally minor surgery can help to elongate the vagina.

13. Pain Management

Pain and cancer are inextricably linked in all our minds. I think that probably one of the greatest fears people have when they are given a cancer diagnosis is that it will, at some point, result in them suffering from unbearable pain for which there is no treatment; this is in general not true and very uncommon. In addition, many people before their diagnosis presume that they cannot have cancer because they have no pain. Ironically this is one of the greatest misconceptions since many cancers unfortunately are not discovered until later than they could have been, specifically because they have not caused any pain. This very much applies to problems in the ovary where there are effectively no pain receptors. It is also true that if one feels pain in a leg or an arm or for instance a finger, then the brain is very good at knowing exactly where the pain is, i.e., if the pain is in your right index finger, the problem is likely to be in your right index finger! It would be inconceivable that the problem would be in your left ring finger. The same does not apply with pain felt in the internal organs, thus the ovary tends not to cause pain unless there is bleeding into it and it rapidly expands or it twists so that its blood supply is cut off; then the pain will be a diffuse pain, usually arising in the lower abdomen. Pain in the uterus is often felt as lower tummy pain, but can also be felt as lower back pain or upper thigh pain. Even more confusingly, the brain can sometimes mistake pain arising from the right for pain felt on the left and vice versa.

In general, when women come to a gynecology clinic with pain, the most common cause is that it is arising from the urinary tract, the most common thing being a urinary tract infection or cystitis. The second most common cause is that it is arising from the bowel and often this can be the condition of irritable bowel syndrome, where there are spasms in the bowel often associated with stress. Pain arising from gynecological organs can be crampy pain associated with periods and bleeding from the uterus. Occasionally, pain can be caused by cysts on the ovary. Two common causes of pain in addition to this are pain caused by infection in the pelvis and pain caused by the condition of endometriosis where the lining of the uterus lies outside the uterus and the pelvis. All of these causes of pain have nothing whatsoever to do with cancer, but can affect the woman who has cancer. In addition, cancer itself can cause pain, either because of the damage that it causes to the tissues in your body or because of damage to nerves supplying those tissues by applying pressure to the nerves or growing into the nerves. The type of treatment you will require will depend upon the type of pain and as you can see from what I have written above, the huge number of things that can cause pain means that the doctor managing your pain requires to ask you a lot of questions to try to tie in your pain with other symptoms. This may even involve giving people a chart so that they can plot how much pain they get, when they get it, and whether it is related to bleeding, urinary function, or bowel function. The rest of this chapter is divided into "systems." By "systems" I mean whether the pain is related to your bowels, to your urinary tract, to your female organs or, finally, whether it is related to pressure on blood vessels.

Bowel System

Constipation

This is very common, particularly where opiate pain killers have been prescribed, e.g., Codeine, morphine, or pethadine, and can result in severe pain in the back passage (rectum). In addition, if there is a lot of impaction of feces, people can get waves of pain as their bowel tries to squeeze out the hard feces without success. This can be treated using a variety of preparations such as laxatives, e.g., Lactulose or Senna granules or, failing this, suppositories can be used. For extreme cases sometimes people have to be admitted to be given enemas to help their bowels move.

Diarrhea

This can be associated with constipation, where there is diarrhea which flows around the constipation. It can also be associated with a tumor pressing on your bowel. Diarrhea is usually managed with Lomotil or Immodium.

Dry Mouth and Throat

This can sometimes be a problem during treatments and can cause much discomfort. Use of mouth washes, sucking on ice cubes, or chewing gum can be helpful, and good oral and dental hygiene are important. If you develop oral thrush, nystatin lozenges can be helpful.

Hiccups

This is a distressing thing to suffer from and usually breathing into a paper bag sorts out the problem, but failing this there are drugs which a doctor can prescribe, e.g., Chlorpromazine or Amphetamines.

Nausea and Vomiting

These are very unpleasant symptoms which can be caused by chemotherapy and radiotherapy, and also by opiate pain killers. These are also common symptoms after people have had surgery. There are now, however, extremely good drugs available, for instance, Ondansitron or Promethazine, which can help with this.

Urinary Tract Problems

Involvement of the urinary tract can cause pain in the lower part of the tummy. It can also cause pain in the small of the back and in the groin. This pain can range from a dull ache to severe "colicky" type pain. The commonest cause of pain is cystitis, which can be caused by infection, and is easily treated with antibiotics. In addition, cystitis can be caused by radiation, and anti-inflammatory drugs can be helpful with this type of pain. Occasionally, pain can be caused by blockage of the ureters (these are the tubes that run between the kidney and bladder) and this can usually be relieved by passing a plastic tube down the blocked ureter. This can either be inserted in the x-ray department and is known as an antegrade stent, or can be inserted in the operating theater via a cystoscope, when it is known as a retrograde stent (Figure 13.1). Occasionally the blockage can only be relieved by a nephrostomy (see Figure 13.1). It is very important to recognize urinary tract infections since occasionally this can also cause infection in the kidney (pyelonephritis). Usually, if this develops you would require to be admitted to hospital for intravenous antibiotics through a drip.

Radiotherapy can sometimes cause pain because of tissue scarring and in addition a burning pain can be felt in the skin. This can usually be helped by 1% hydrocortisone cream or local anesthetic cream.

Chemotherapy can cause pain and there is a condition called "peripheral neuropathy." This is where there is tingling and numbness in the fingers and toes. This almost always gets better over time, but can be much helped by drug therapy. In addition, chemotherapy can cause inflammation in the mouth and throat, gullet, and stomach, and all of these can be helped by various lozenges, drinks, etc.

Lymphedema

This is a troublesome condition which occurs when the lymph fluid leaks out of the blood vessels and causes uncomfortable swelling. Lymph fluid is normally collected in channels called lymphatic channels and is transferred back into the blood stream. After removal of lymph nodes, coupled often with radiotherapy, there is damage to the lymphatic channels and they are no longer able to transfer the lymph back into the blood stream. The effect of the lymph

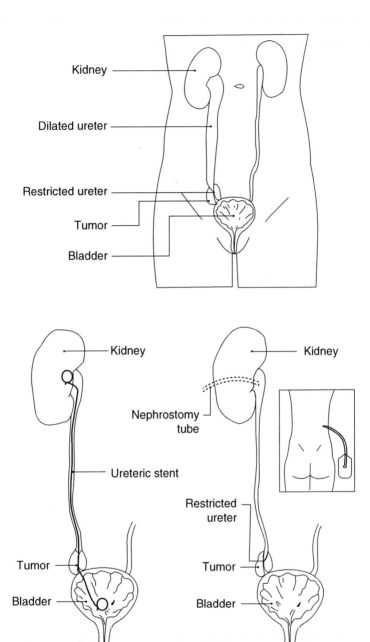

Figure 13.1. Methods of treating urinary tract obstruction

being unable to get back into the blood stream is to cause localized swelling. Unfortunately, because of the localized swelling, the swollen area is prone to low-grade infections. Sometimes your doctor will give you low-dose antibiotics to treat this and will almost certainly suggest certain types of bandaging, and occasionally intermittent pressure boots (Figure 13.2). They will also suggest that you should elevate the effected area. The elevation encourages all the fluid to track back into the blood stream.

Painkillers

These are also known as analgesic drugs. There are a huge number of drugs, which can relieve pain. These have different ways of working. Some of them are anti-inflammatory and some are opiate type drugs. The drug, which will be selected for you will be appropriate to your pain. It is important to say that among this wide variety these drugs come in differing strengths and clearly

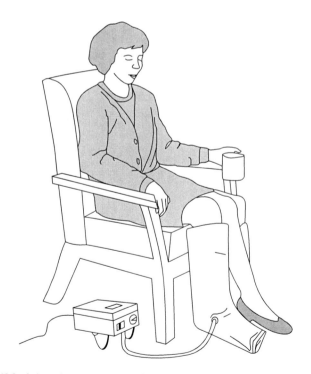

Figure 13.2. An intermittent positive pressure boot can reduce lymph volume

your doctor will want to discover what is the best drug and best strength for you. This may change over time, requiring changes of drugs and changes in strengths of drugs. In addition to pain killers, antidepressants can also be used for getting rid of pain. Often people are worried about taking these because they feel that the drug has been given as an antidepressant. In fact, when anti-depressants are given as pain killers, they are given in a dose which would not have any affect on depression. They do, however, have an effect on the nerves which are transmitting the pain and this is how they work. Steroids can also be beneficial, since they reduce inflammation and swelling. The chapter on complementary therapies deals exhaustively with complementary approaches to pain. You may, if you are getting problems with pain, find that you are referred to a chronic pain specialist or the palliative care specialist. Both of these groups of specialists are highly experienced in managing pain symptoms.

It is vitally important that you do tell your doctor or specialist nurse if you are suffering from pain, because it is highly likely that they will be able to help your pain by one route or another. In my own experience it is very rare to find patients with gynecological cancer in pain for which we have no treatment.

14. Complementary Therapies

This chapter discusses the pros and cons of various treatments. It is divided into separate sections on hypnotherapy, acupuncture, homeopathy, meditation, spiritual healing, and Reike. In addition, there is a section on psychotherapy and counseling.

I have not discussed diet in this book, not because I do not think it important, but rather because most people know the value of good balanced healthy diet, with a mixture of food types. There is a great emphasis in the lay press on eating one's way to being disease-free, which is nonsense. It is, however, true that one can eat one's way to ill health, while unfortunately a good diet does not protect one from ill health. There is certainly no evidence that meat avoidance protects against cancer and in the time around your operation where blood may be lost red meat can be very beneficial: a steak is equivalent to three iron tablets and better for you.

Hypnotherapy

This technique was originally described by the French physician Mesmer, hence the other name for the hypnotic state, "mesmerism." Since its discovery nearly 200 years ago it has always remained on the fringes of medical practice. It has undoubtedly gained a variable reputation, partly down to the antics of stage hypnotists. While there is no doubting the entertainment properties of the technique, these have overshadowed and undermined the potential of hypnosis for treatment of a wide variety of conditions. I myself have taught many patients the ability to self-hypnotize, thus allowing treatment of phobias (needles, flying, etc.), inability to sleep, wound pain, menopausal flushes, and many other things. The other problem for hypnosis in terms of acceptance within the medical profession is a lack of research data to support it, although this is now improving. When I was practicing in Glasgow I used to teach self-hypnosis for vaginal pain following childbirth. At first I was not sure how successful this was, until husbands started bringing me bottles of whisky and boxes of cigars! This may not have been scientific evidence but I found it reasonably convincing that I was doing some good. Hypnosis also has the benefit that for those that it does not help it rarely does harm. I regularly hypnotize myself, particularly if I cannot sleep or before lectures to big audiences, and it gives me a feeling of calm before "facing the crowd." Most of us require three to four sessions to learn the technique, the first lasting an hour and the others 30 minutes.

The other great fear generated by stage hypnotists is that the technique allows others to enter into the deeper private parts of your mind and somehow to gain control over you. In general, no hypnotist can make people do that which they have no desire to do. There is no doubting that hypnosis is a powerful tool and that it needs to be done by someone you know and trust, a trained hypnotherapist, doctor, dentist, psychologist, or yourself.

In Glasgow in the 1980s there was a famous stage hypnotist, Robert Halpern, who during his show appeared to gain complete control of about 50 people in an audience of 1,500 and make these poor unfortunates do all sorts of ridiculous and entertaining things. Many of my patients who had seen this show used to ask how I could possibly say that hypnosis did not give enormous power to the hypnotist. Having seen the show myself I could tell them that it started by Halpern using a well-recognized method for testing people's capacity for hypnosis (in general, most people are hypnotizable, lack of concentration, cynicism, and old age being the main factors stopping you). He used a technique where he asked the audience to clasp their hands together. He then told them that their hands would get tighter and tighter together as he counted from one to ten. With this a high proportion of his audience showed the start of the hypnotic response but only a few (50 out of 1,500) followed through to the point where they could no longer release their hands. This group of 50 was then invited onto the stage if they wanted their hands released, which of course they could not until the end of the show! The group on the stage was then induced into full trance state. The remaining 1,450 people had consciously withdrawn from the hypnotic process. It is reasonable to presume that there will always be a few exhibitionists in every audience!

How does hypnosis work? Nobody knows exactly how it works, but it appears to be a method of allowing access to, and control over, one's subconscious and deep subconscious. The conscious means that of which we are aware. The subconscious is the activity bubbling away below the surface that we usually only experience in dreams and under the influence of certain drugs. The deep subconscious is that part of the brain controlling processes like beating of the heart, breathing, and other bodily functions that in general we do not "thinkingly" control. Normally, our conscious self cannot gain entry to, or control over, our subconscious or deep subconscious. There are exceptions to this, for example, you breathe without thinking, but can, if you wish, hold your breath. You cannot, however, control your own heart rate. Hypnosis allows access to this part of the brain. Examples of this would be that under self-hypnosis you can alter your pulse at will, or a dentist hypnotizing you before tooth extraction can stop you salivating and bleeding from the socket. I myself have carried out a number of surgical procedures without anesthetic under hypnosis with the patient feeling nothing. Figure 14.1 shows a schematic representation of how hypnosis works, allowing access of the conscious to the deeper part of the mind.

- Conscious
- Subconscious
- Deep subconscious (including pulse rate)

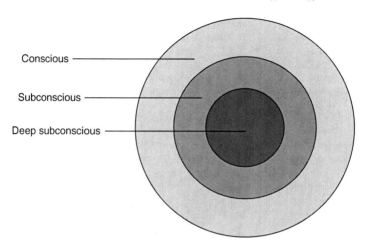

Figure 14.1. Schematic representation of the mind

I myself select patients who I believe may be suitable candidates for hypnotherapy on the basis of their age, strength of personality, and apparent capacity for concentration. Much at odds with what you might think, the best candidates are usually from childhood to middle age and the stronger the personality, the better. If you are an older patient you may have got to a cynical stage in life, making you a poor candidate. None of these criteria is hard and fast and certainly there is little to lose and much to gain by trying.

It is possible to use the Halpern technique of hand clasping to assess your hypnotizability. Another method is to tell you to close your eyes and that there is a large weight on top of your head and it is getting heavier as I count to ten. I then observe to see if your head starts to nod. In general, it is better to go straight to trying to hypnotize you.

Most people want to know what it will feel like when they are hypnotized. This is not something that one can easily describe. It does, however, feel slightly "other worldly," a bit like the "removed" feeling one gets after taking a sleep-inducing drug. It taps into that place where one is neither awake nor asleep. When you are hypnotized you can talk, hear everything that is going on around you, and you can wake up whenever you want, although most people usually do not want to! I always tell people if they feel an itch, or feel uncomfortable, they can move about, scratch themselves, or whatever.

Those patients wishing to go ahead are brought back to a clinic where an hour will have been allotted for the first visit and probably half an hour for each subsequent visit. You will be asked to sit in an easy chair or lie on a couch and firstly to do some gentle breathing exercises. These comprise imagining that there is a candle in front of you. If you are somebody who breathes through your nose you will be asked to breathe in through your nose and out through your mouth. If you are a mouth breather you will be asked to breathe in and out through your mouth. The breath out, whichever way you breathe, will last to the count of 10 seconds and should be done as if you were slowly blowing out a candle. Doing this for 1 or 2 minutes is always very relaxing. You will then be asked to tense various muscle groups and let them relax. I usually start with toes and tell people to tense their toes and relax. Then I ask them to tense their calf muscles and relax, tense their thigh muscles and relax, tense their abdominal muscles and relax. By this time you can feel yourself sinking into the bed. We finish with you tensing the chest muscles and relaxing them, lifting your shoulders and letting them relax, and finally screwing up your face and letting it relax.

I then ask you to concentrate on a point which is above and just behind you, enough to make a slight strain on the eyes. I then tell you I am going to count to ten and as I do so you will feel your eye lids getting heavier and heavier, to the point where you will have to let them close. You should continue to breathe like you are blowing out the candle. As I count to ten I am watching your eyelids, which usually start to flicker and then close. This is usually an irresistible feeling, quite pleasant and not to be resisted.

I then ask you to imagine that you are on top of a hill, the hill is covered with beautiful lush grass, and you can smell the grass. In Scotland I used to suggest heather. Overhead is a bright blue sky with the sun shining and a light breeze cooling your face. At the bottom of the hill is a brook, which you can hear babbling in the distance. I am going to count to ten and you are going to walk down the hill. As you do so you will go deeper and deeper into the hypnotic state. I then count to ten: one, two, three, four, five, you are now half way down the hill and feeling more and more deeply asleep, more and more relaxed, six, seven, eight, nine, and ten. Now you are at the bottom of the hill and feeling beautifully relaxed. This process of going down the hill can be repeated two or three times depending upon the patient. I always look for the various signs that it is going well: breathing changes from the chest moving up and down to your tummy moving instead.

Occasionally, I may think that the patient is just pretending so as not to hurt my feelings, if this is the case we start again using a different technique.

There are many ways of inducing a hypnotic trance; all however utilize similar techniques to those described above. Others include walking down a beach, or counting out loud backwards from 100 by subtracting three, i.e. 100, 97, 94, etc.

Once you are in a deep trance various approaches can be taken depending upon the initial complaint and the goal of the therapy.

In offering hypnotherapy to patients I have used it for relief of wound pain, relief of tummy and groin pain, relief of menopausal symptoms in women unable to take hormone replacement therapy, management of needle phobia, and as a replacement for general anesthetic. I have also used it as a confidence builder. Its use as an alternative to general anesthesia is, in general, not warranted, since it is extremely time-consuming to get a subject to this level of confidence in the technique.

At the end of the hypnotic session you will be taught how to pre program yourself so that you can get into the trance more quickly the next time. I use a process where I press my thumb against my index finger and count one, then on my middle finger and count two, then on my ring finger and count three, then on my pinkie and count four on the inner surface and five on the outer. By doing this in future I induce the same trance in about 10 seconds! You will then be told that in future you cannot be hypnotized by anybody other than a doctor, a dentist, a psychologist or somebody you know and trust including yourself. This will mean you can go and watch Halpern with complete impunity!

You will then be told that when you wake up you will feel beautifully relaxed and refreshed and that you should count back from five to one in your head and slowly come back awake. This you will duly do, usually with some reluctance since the feeling is so good!

I will illustrate some of the uses from my own experience: Many years ago I went to a respected hypnotherapist because I smoked 20 cigarettes per day, I was asthmatic, and I was two stones overweight. I was hypnotized and once in a trance my hypnotherapist utilized a schemata derived from Hindu/Bhuddist thinking. In this you are asked which you see as the most important part of you, your face, your chest, your gut, or your groin. These relate to your chakras. We all often describe people as operating on a gut level, or having a big heart or being driven by their groin! For me my dominant chakra is in my chest. The hypnotherapist taught me to imagine my chest opening up like a flower. Once open, it was bathed in bright light and my asthmatic lungs washed with pure water! After this I was asked to let the power in my chest flow out of it like a fountain. Once I could feel this I was asked to close the flower down and to make this newly recognized power flow through my arms down to my finger tips. Following this I was asked to describe where I most liked to smoke. I described the terrace in front of my family house on one of the islands off the west coast of Scotland (Bute). From there I was taken to a room, my Room 101. In it there was a television and a door. I was in the television and in the room. The me in the television was me 20 years later. By this time I had developed bronchitis and could not breathe without an oxygen mask and I was wracked with terrible coughing fits. The hypnotherapist gave me a choice either to be in the television or to walk through a door which had just opened. Through the door was the fresh air and sunshine of Bute and being a nonsmoker. I started to walk to the door, but hesitated at the door; the hypnotherapist asked what I wanted to do? Be in Room 101 as a smoker or in the fresh air as a nonsmoker; this time I walked through the door and have not smoked a cigarette in 8 years. I did not put on weight, and in fact, I lost two stones. This and saying no to cigarettes proved very easy. Any time I was tempted to overeat or smoke I would self-hypnotize and utilizing the power of the chest chakra I would have no difficulty in what I can only describe as pushing away (psychologically) the offending item.

I do a lot of lecturing to medical students, other doctors, and patient groups. Before lectures where there is a big audience, there are few who will not admit to feelings of nervousness. When I am sitting at the front of the audience just a few minutes before going to the podium I will self-hypnotize using the quick induction technique described above. I then imagine the power in my chest chakra flowing through my arms into my hands and into my fingers. I instantly feel relaxed and tell myself that the lecture will go well. I then count back from five to one and feel relaxed and confident!

I have illustrated above how you can be hypnotized and some of its uses. There are innumerable problems that it can be used for. One of the biggest difficulties is in finding a respectable practitioner, but personal recommendation or using a member or the Society of Medical and Dental Hypnotherapists or a psychologist is usually a route to being safely taught how to self-hypnotize.

Acupuncture/Shiatsu

This is an ancient form of Chinese medicine based on meridians. There are two schools of practice: one is the traditional Chinese method, which sees the body in holistic terms. The needles may be heated and herbs applied to the top of the needles. Traditionally, these needles were reused and, as you can imagine, with the risks of hepatitis B and HIV, strict sterilization is now needed if needles are to be reused. Many non-Chinese doctors, nurses, and physiotherapists now use acupuncture usually as a form of pain relief. Modern medicine does not wholly understand how the acupuncture needle points work.

Shiatsu and acupuncture are based on the same points in the body. These theories arose in the Far East in Japan and China and are based on a theory of "energy lines" in the body. These can be affected either by pressure or by the use of needles. Shiatsu is a form of massage utilizing these meridians by pressure, and acupuncture involves the insertion of needles.

Acupuncture has become very popular for pain relief both with doctors practicing Chinese medicine and chronic pain specialists. In the UK and the USA many pain specialists who usually have started their training as specialists in anesthesia have learnt acupuncture and incorporated this into their pain relief practice. I know that two of my own colleagues, one a pain specialist and the other a gynecologist, use it regularly to help their patients cope with pain. The needle is placed at a site distant from where the pain is according to the meridian principle, e.g., pain in the upper part of the mouth is relieved by a needle in the ear lobe.

There is however no doubt that many patients have gained great relief through this method as well as enhanced feelings of well-being. We do know that the needles release the body's endorphins. These are opiate-like substances produced in all of us, which are not dissimilar in chemical structure to the opiates, e.g., Morphine, which are administered as pain killers. What is not understood is how pressure in one place induces pain relief in a distant part of the body, e.g., the relief of nausea from pressure over the wrist.

Homeopathy

This is a very popular form of alternative therapy which utilizes a system of medicines derived from plants, minerals, and animal products. In scientific terms, the theory behind homeopathy is counterintuitive. The homeopathist, who may well be a qualified doctor, will take your history and take into account your physical and emotional needs. They will then identify a medicament that if given to a healthy person would give them your symptoms. The remedy is then diluted down up to nine times. The more the dilution, the stronger is the expected effect; this is the part that the rationalist has to find counterintuitive. Not withstanding that we do not understand how it works, many patients seem to derive great benefit from these treatments. In the medical journals the debate continues much as it has for the last 200 years as to the effectiveness of these treatments. For my money, if something has been around for that amount of time there must be something in it, even if we do not understand it! Recently, there has been a much greater effort on the part of the homeopathic community to subject their medications to trials, much as standard drugs are. These suggest that some remedies do sometimes produce the desired effect! In my own practice I do sometimes suggest Arnica for wound healing and regularly refer to a colleague who is a registered homeopathist. In the UK there are two homeopathic hospitals: one in London and one in Glasgow.

Alexander Technique

I include mention of this technique for completeness. It is an approach to the way we stand, hold ourselves, walk, and sit. It is of great benefit to those suffering from neck and joint pain, breathing disorders, and stress-related disorders. It is particularly popular with musicians, especially violinists, who by the nature of their job place their bodies in unnatural positions. It also makes people usually gain an inch or two in height once they have learnt the technique – maybe I should try it myself – I could certainly do with gaining vertical inches rather than horizontal ones!

Massage, Reflexology, Meditation, Yoga, and Spiritual Healing

The placing of all of these different techniques under one banner is not intended as any insult or diminution in any particular one. They are however all a bit like a Venn diagram – I do not know if you remember them from school maths (see Figure 14.2). Massage is a system of stroking, kneading, and pressing different areas of the body to relieve stress and strain; it is particularly good for muscle and joint pains. I doubt if there is anybody who does not feel better after massage.

Reflexology again originated in the Far East and is a form of foot/hand massage again relying on meridians for an effect distant from the foot.

To my mind meditation, self-hypnosis, and the mental side of yoga are all one and the same. There are various exercises whereby one can gain access to the subconscious, the inner self. Chapter 16 on spiritual aspects also deals with this. Yoga is very popular. It was invented in India and is a method of harmonizing mind, body and emotions, using posture, breathing, movement, and meditation to achieve feelings of well-being.

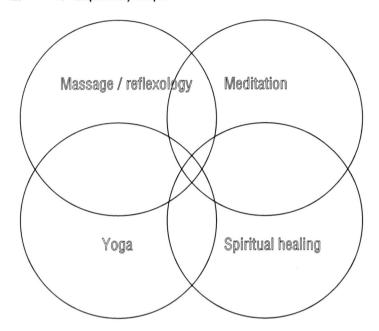

Figure 14.2. Venn diagram

Psychotherapy

There are a number of different approaches to psychology. Historically psychology started at the beginning of the 20th century with Freud. C.G. Jung (Figure 14.3) was originally a "disciple" of Freud before breaking with him and developing his own approaches. These have continued to be developed and are currently taught at many places, among them the Jungian Institute at Kusnacht on the shores of the Zurichsee (see Figure 14.4). Adler followed with a different approach again. Modern psychologists will have learnt a medley of these approaches. There is also a "crossover" between orthodox psychotherapists and some complementary therapists who have also been trained in aspects of psychotherapy.

A form of psychotherapy known as logotherapy has also become popular. This was invented by Dr. Vicktor Frankl, a doctor who was imprisoned in Auschwitz concentration camp during the Second World War and survived. His principal observation was that the few who survived the death camp had a unifying feature, namely a belief that they were here for a purpose. Logotherapy is a psychological method of helping patients discover this side of themselves.

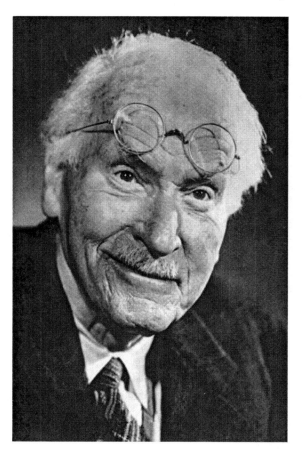

Figure 14.3. CG Jung

Counseling

There are a plethora of counseling services available to people these days. How much a person wants to talk about their condition varies from one individual to another. To my mind, the meeting together of groups who have suffered similarly, perhaps with a counseling facilitator, seems to help many. I have no doubt that many people are genuinely helped by counselors, but I also have no doubt that we live in an age where we are on the opposite swing of the pendulum from the "stiff upper lip" approach, where we were encouraged to not talk about anything. We have now arrived at perhaps a time of overintense "navel-gazing"

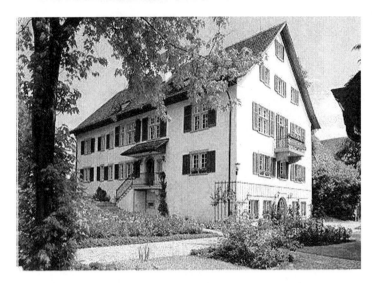

Figure 14.4. The Jungian Institute, Küsnacht, Switzerland

and a compulsion to talk about our problems, which does not suit everyone. I am sure that somewhere in between, which is tailored to the individual, is best!

As you will detect, of the complementary therapies discussed, the only one which I have personally practiced is hypnotherapy. I have developed a network of colleagues to whom I refer to for the other treatments. What people select is largely a matter of their personal preference, though some do not want any of these things, but most will find that at least one appeals to them.

15. Bereavement/Grief

Bereavement is by definition the process we go through when we suffer loss of something or someone very special to us. In terms of this book it therefore applies to women diagnosed with cancer who are coping with the loss that this entails and to the relatives of the minority of women who will sadly succumb to their disease.

At the time of diagnosis there is an enormous range of emotions at play. These are denial, anger, grief, depression, aggression, numbness, etc. There is no doubting that at that first consultation numbness and disbelief will be the strongest emotions, as well as the thought of why me? I have done nothing to deserve this, I have eaten healthily, not smoked, not drunk, it cannot be true. However, over the next few days/weeks when the management plan is clarified, there is the coping with loss of organs if surgery is planned, and this may involve loss of fertility or feelings of loss of womanhood, and a true bereavement process unfolds. If this is the first major illness you have encountered, there will also be that loss of invincibility. I think we all feel invincible, it will never happen to us, until it does – and that is a terrible shock. Anger may center on why me? Why have I been dealt this hand of cards? If you are religious you may wonder why God has allowed this to happen to you?

Traditionally, bereavement has been seen in the stepwise progression suggested by Elizabeth Kubla-Ross, from denial to anger to grief to bewilderment to depression to acceptance and hope, with a new way of being. Things will never be the same again, but life can go on albeit differently. A different model encompassing the same emotions is the "tapestry of bereavement or a landscape of grief." This model was taught to me by my friend Gary Bradley, the founder and chairman of the Westminster Bereavement Association. The analogy here is with a picture. When you buy a picture there are various features of the picture which you may have noticed, but as the picture hangs on the wall you notice, over time, different aspects of the picture until after some time you may hardly notice the picture at all, even though it is still there. You may however move the picture and it instantly becomes more visible.

↓ Denial	D
↓ Anger	A
↓ Bewilderment/bargaining	B
↓ Depression	D
↓ Acceptance	A
↓ Hope	H

D Denial

A Anger

B Bewilderment/Bargaining

D Depression

A Acceptance

H Hope

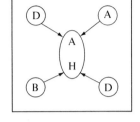

Figure 15.1. Sketch of the "Tapestry of Bereavement/Landscape of Grief"

The picture then is as shown in the sketch in Figure 15.1, where the various emotions crop up not in any particular order but more randomly, with some predominating at one point and others at another. Over time, acceptance and hope arrive and then the other parts of the tapestry fade and while they do not disappear the tapestry becomes your new reality.

This may all appear somewhat negative, but one of the amazing and heartening things which many people say to me is that their cancer diagnosis finally gave them great inner strength and that they went on to do things that they know they would not otherwise have done – this is the concept of winning through losing – a very difficult place to get to, but something that can be genuinely empowering for the individual.

For those who lose a spouse, relative, or close friend the same range of emotions will occur and the tapestry is similar. The "tapestry" by its flexibility and its ability to fade and then come back into focus may be a useful model for you to think around.

This process, particularly when one arrives at hope and acceptance, ties in with the Venn diagram of psychology, spirituality, and religion described in the next chapter. These are the areas that most will choose to further explore.

16. Spiritual Approaches to Living with Cancer

You may consider it brave, foolhardy, presumptuous, or just plain not appropriate for a doctor like me to even enter into this subject. My reason for including a chapter on this subject is that over the last 10–15 years I have had the privilege to look after a large number of women who have either been cured of their cancer or have lived with their cancer for a long time before succumbing to the disease, I have become quite convinced that religion and spirituality allow people to cope better with their disease than those who see things in strictly secular, non-religious terms. Spirituality is used as meaning the attempt to experience a sense of the transcendental independent of religion. I would not dream of suggesting that I think that those with religion live longer with their disease, but I do believe that particularly for those who are living with cancer many of them do "live better." You may think when you start this chapter that "I'm somebody who's not religious, not spiritual so there's no point in reading this," or that you are religious and once again, therefore, there is not much point in reading it because how does one change the way that one is! I think it is also important that I state here at the start of this chapter that I have no agenda whatsoever to proselytize for any specific religion. I myself could have been regarded as a non-practicing Christian for the first 35 years of my life and for the last few I have practiced, or at least tried to practice, Christianity in a liberal Anglo-Catholic tradition. I do also have a keen interest in Eastern Orthodoxy, in particular in aspects concerned with Christian mysticism. I impart this information not through any desire to suggest that what I do is better than what anybody else does, but merely to be clear in my own position. Ironically, it has been the juxtaposition of looking after patients with cancer and *human immunodeficiency virus* (HIV), watching their coping mechanisms and having to develop some of my own, coupled with a brief but severe bout of personal illness and difficulty, which propelled me along my own personal route.

One of the things I have been struck by is the common ground between the great religions: Christianity, Judaism, Islam, Hinduism, and Buddhism. Mandalas are found in many of these religions (see Figure 16.1). To my mind, in health terms, the type of religious belief is unimportant. What does matter is the belief itself. Apart from the moral code, one of the unifying themes of all religions is that they all have a monastic element, and for that small group of "holy people," be they men or women, there is a unifying feature of "seeking the light." Until I read around this area, I had never realized that the common saying to "see the light" was a reference to that other-worldly light. The Greek and

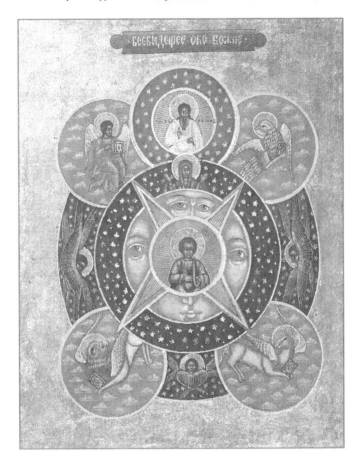

Figure 16.1. Picture of Christian Mandala: the all seeing eye of God

Russian hesychast monk enters via ascetism into a trance-like state to see the light. Renaissance art obsesses with "the Light," the white dove, the holy spirit of the Trinity. The Sufi Muslim seeks the light as does the Buddhist yogi. This light is that which is sought by the holy of all religions. That holy is spelt with an "H," but, it could just as easily be spelt with a "Wh," wholly. I cannot believe that all these holy people, whatever their tradition, are seeing different "lights".

Surely, it can be no coincidence that many of those patients who have had near-death experiences describe seeing a light and that they felt as if they were going on a journey into the light.

I have had patients from all of these belief systems and there is undoubtedly a common thread running through all of the world's major religions. When it comes to living with cancer they all seem to have the capacity to provide reassurance and hope in equal measure to each other. It is noteworthy that hospitals historically, certainly in the Western tradition, grew out of monasteries where there was a belief in tending to the physical, emotional, and religious well-being of those being cared for. To my mind, this is one of the failings of modern medicine, that as we have got far better at achieving higher cure rates, and have much more to offer as every year goes by, we have left the care of the spiritual side of the patient behind almost as a matter of irrelevance. Worse than this, it is almost impossible to enter the arena of religion with your patient without a serious danger of being seen as a proselytizer, something which I have absolutely no intention or desire to be seen as.

I have been interested for many years in the work of Carl Gustav Jung, the famous Swiss psychologist. I do think that Jung saw the link between psychology and religion and his insights came partly through dream analysis. Jung coined the term "individuation," by which he meant that process by which a person becomes a psychological individual, i.e., a separate, indivisible unity or "whole," meaning that the person has come to selfhood or self-realization. He firmly believed that people only got to this place and became in psychoanalytical terms "mature" when, for most individuals, they passed the age of 40. Jung's view on dreams is much more interesting than any dictionary definition: "The dream is the little hidden door in the innermost and most secret recesses of the psyche. ... All consciousness separates; but in dreams we put on the likeness of that more universal, truer, more eternal man dwelling in the darkness of primordial night." Jung believed in the collective subconscious. The subconscious is that place which can be entered by achieving a dream-like or trance-like state. Many religious ceremonies achieve this with the combination of ritual, chanting, and a mixture of sights, sounds, and smells, which have the capacity to induce a semi-hypnotic state. The current obsession with yoga is almost certainly tapping into something similar. Chapter 14 deals with hypnotherapy, meditation, etc.

I always find it interesting that when you read works by religious authors they always feel that any reference to hypnotherapy or hypnosis as having aspects bearing on religion is somehow an insult to that religion. Conversely, the psychologist wishes to avoid entering the arena of religion as the forbidden zone. I have never really understood why entering into the subconscious, be it via a hypnotherapy session, seeing a psychologist, or partaking in a religious ceremony which allows one access to one's god, should be seen in anything other than positive terms.

It is noteworthy that when Jung was questioned in public about whether he believed in God himself he replied, "I do not believe in God...." And then paused. After what seemed an age he continued, "I know." Ironically Richard Dawkins in his book "The God Delusion" pillories CG Jung as 100% theist i.e. believer in God. The irony comes on page 40 of Dawkin's book where he concluds his summary of Einstein's views on God. Einstein stated "to sense that behind anything that can be experienced there is something that our mind cannot grasp and whose beauty and sublimity reaches us only indirectly and as a feeble reflection, this is religiousness, in this sense I am religious". Dawkins follows this quote by himself saying "in this sense I am religious with the

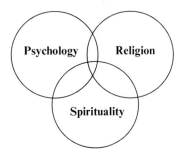

Figure 16.2.

reservation that cannot grasp does not have to mean forever ungraspable". Reading Jung, I would dare to argue that Jung's and Dawkins' views strongly coincide. Of course, Dawkins goes on to say that "religion" implies "supernatural". Many would contest this assertion feeling that religion was their chosen path to their god. My own feeling is that as per Figure 16.2 the important thing is to find the route that suits you be it theistic or atheistic.

In addition to the mainstream religions there are also individuals who are spiritual healers who may come from shamanistic or pagan belief systems or utilize aspects of Buddhism or Christianity. I personally refer those patients who are interested in a spiritual approach and who have no religion to a spiritual healer of the Buddhist tradition; he has often worked wonders. For those who are lapsed from their original religion they may wish to revisit it. For those who are less interested, the help of counselors or psychologists to find the inner self and inner peace again can be helpful.

The great difficulty is how to get into the subject in the first place with your patients and this is something, by my own experience, which is only sometimes possible and almost always when I have truly got to know the patient. Even then, entering the discussion can be fraught with difficulty, again relating back to the danger of being seen as a proselytizer. The irony is that if one finds that somebody has no religion, then the route is certainly not to suggest that they start going to church or their local temple, but rather that they go down the psychological route. The enormous success of Deepak Chopra's books, Mind Body Healing etc., is ample testimony to the unmet need here.

I have put some suggested further reading (pages 131) for those who wish to explore this area further. The venn diagram (Fig 16.2) shows the crossover between spirituality, psychology, and religion demonstrating separateness as well as the crossover.

17. Conclusion

It may seem strange to finish a book such as this with some conclusions. However, the book started with some key aims:

1. Most important to me is that you have gained accurate information. This is not easy in our current times with masses of internet information available, much of which is highly dubious.

2. When you are told that you have cancer, you (along with everybody else) will have a thought that "I'm going to die very soon." This is virtually never the case – the vast majority of people are in cusps A and B, i.e., "cured" or "living with cancer," NOT preterminal (cusp C), or dying (cusp D) (see 4-cusp picture in Chapter 3).

3. All of you will experience grief/bereavement after the diagnosis, although most of you will live for long periods of time after this and the majority will be cured. The landscape of grief may prove to be a useful model for you (see landscape picture on page 116).

4. You can see the different strands of orthodox and complementary medicines and how in each of these spheres some things will be right for you and others not, but you, in conjunction with your doctors, nurses, and therapists will find what is right for you in the knowledge that you know what is available.

5. If you are of a religious/spiritual frame of mind you persevere with this, expand it, and if you are not, you either go down the route of psychological intervention (either by the orthodox route of clinical psychology or the complementary route, e.g., hypnotherapy), or if this is not your way, try practical approaches. The three patients who wrote pieces typify, by pure chance on my part, these different approaches (see Venn diagram on page 119).

6. The diagnosis of cancer changes your life and that of your family and close friends for ever, but to quote Maggie Keswick Jencks again "above all, what matters is not to lose the joy of living in the fear of dying."

Suggested Further Reading

1. Lawrence van der Post, *Jung and the story of our time*. Vintage 2002.
2. C G Jung, *The Undiscovered Self*. Routledge 1996.
3. *The way of a Pilgrim* translated and annotated Glebb Pocrowsky. Dart and Longman Todd 2001.
4. C G Jung, *Memories, Dream, Reflections*. Fontana Press 1995.
5. C G Jung, *Modern Man in Search of a Soul*. Routledge *2001*.
6. Jennifer Lash, *On pilgrimage*. Bloomsbury 1998.
7. Arnold Mindel, *The Shaman's Body*. Harper San Franscisco 1993.
8. Thomas Merton, *The Intimate Merton*. Lion 2002.
9. Soyal Rinpoche, *The Tibetan Book of Living and Dying*. Random House 1992.
10. Deepak Chopra, *Quantum Healing*. Bantam 1989.
11. Bernie Siegel, *Love, Medicine and Miracles*. Arrow 1988.
12. Laurens Van Der Post, *The Seed and the Sower*. Hogarth Press 1963.
13. John Diamond. *Snake Dance*.
14. Cassandra Marks, *Homeopathy: A Step by Step Guide*. Element Books 1997.
15. Michael Geerin-Tosh, *Living proof, a medical mutiny*. Scribner 2002.
16. www.jrsmithgynaecology.com: this provides a comprehensive description of all the operations described in this book with art work by Dee MacLean.
17. Viktor Frankl *Man's Search For Meaning*. Ebury Press, Random House, London 1959, 2004. www.viktorfrankl.org.

Glossary

Appendix:	"Worm-like" structure in the bowel neck of the womb
Ascites	Fluid in the abdominal cavity
Cervix:	neck of the womb
CIN:	cervical intraepithelial neoplasia "ectomy": removal of an organ, e.g., appendicectomy
Endometrium:	lining of the womb
Fallopian tube:	the "tube" between the uterus and ovary
FIGO:	Federation International Gynaecologie Oncologie, an international Committee, who advise on 'staging' of disease – see below
HPV:	human papilloma virus
Lymph nodes:	glands which are situated alongside blood vessels
Metastasis (plural = metastases):	cancer, which has spread from its primary (original) site, also known as secondary cancer
Omentum:	fatty structure hanging from the large bowel
"ostomy":	to fashion a hole in an organ, e.g., colostomy: to fashion a hole in the colon (large bowel)
Ovaries:	the organs which produce eggs; when they stop working is when the menopause arrives
Parametrium stage:	the area lying lateral to the cervix i.e. alongside the cervix
Primary cancer:	the place where the cancer has started
Staging	The amount that a cancer has spread. It is always divided into I, II, III, IV. Stage I being earliest, i.e. not spread. Stage IV is latest, i.e. spread widely
Secondary cancer:	cancer which has spread from its original, primary site, also known as metastases
Uterus:	womb
VAIN:	vaginal intraepithelial neoplasia – a precancerous condition of the vaginal skin
VIN:	vulval intraepithelial neoplasia – a precancerous condition of the vulva
Vulva:	the skin on the outside of the vagina, encompassing the labia majora (hair-bearing skin), the labia minora (the inner lips) and the clitoris

Index

LaVergne, TN USA
13 October 2010
200548LV00007B/1/P